# Environment and Health: A Holistic Approach

The international symposium Man...Health...Environment, held in Luxembourg 3–5 March 1988, was the closing event of the European Year of the Environment (EYE).

The official representative of the Luxembourg Ministry of the Environment for all EYE matters was Paul Weber. The organisation, coordination and secretariat of the one hundred Luxembourg EYE projects, including the symposium, was entrusted by the Ministry to E.J. Lorang (LUX CONFERENCE s.c.).

The Scientific Programme of the Conference was entrusted to the International Society for Research on Civilization Diseases and on Environment (SIRMCE).

This book, based on the conference, was organised, edited, translated, and produced by POPLAR s.c. of Brussels.

# Environment and Health: A Holistic Approach

*Edited by*

ROBERT KRIEPS
*Minister of the Environment*
*Grand Duchy of Luxembourg*

*based on the conference*

MAN . . . HEALTH . . . ENVIRONMENT

*sponsored by the*

*Luxembourg Ministries of Environment and Health*
*the Commission of the European Communities*
*and the World Health Organization*

Avebury
Aldershot · Brookfield USA · Hong Kong · Singapore · Sydney

Except in the cases of Mr Brinkhorst of the Commission of the European Communities, Dr Kreisel of the World Health Organization, Dr Tockert of International Physicians for the Prevention of Nuclear War and Dr Tolba of the United Nations Environment Programme, the views expressed by the authors in this book are attributable only to them in a personal capacity and not to any institutions.

Published by

Avebury
Gower Publishing Company Limited
Gower House
Croft Road
Aldershot
Hants GU11 3HR
England

Gower Publishing Company
Old Post Road
Brookfield
Vermont 05036
USA



**British Library Cataloguing in Publication Data**
Man -- Health -- Environment conference
Environment and health: a holistic approach: based on the conference Man -- Health -- Conference sponsored by the Luxembourg Ministries of Environment and Health, the commission of the European Communities, and the World Health Organisation
1. Environmental Health
I. Title II. Krieps, Robert, 1922--
363.7

**ISBN 0 566 07050 2**

Printed and bound in Great Britain by
Antony Rowe Limited, Chippenham, Wiltshire

# Contents

# Tables

# Figures

# Notes on contributors

**Professor Günter Altner,** Dr Theol. and Dr Rer. Nat., teaches at the Pädagogische Hochschule of Koblenz, Federal Republic of Germany (FRG) and is the co-editor of several Protestant theological publications. He was the co-founder, in 1977, of the Institute for Applied Ecology in Freiburg. From 1979 to 1982, Professor Altner was a member of a commission of the Bundestag on future nuclear energy policies and in 1982 he founded the Günter Altner Foundation, in Heidelberg, to promote ecological and peace-oriented research projects.

**Dr Aloys Bernatzky** studied philosophy and theology, garden and landscape architecture, urban architecture, geography, botany and ethnography, and has worked for forty years in governmental departments, on town planning and environment protection, in Frankfurt am Main, Darmstadt and Wiesbaden, Federal Republic of Germany. He has done research on city ecology, the influence of green areas on city climate, tree surgery, and the influence of electromagnetic waves on biological systems, and is the author of several books on tree ecology, conservation and green area management.

**Mme Huguette Bouchardeau** is a Member of Parliament and was Minister of the Environment and the Quality of Life in France from 1984 to 1986, after having been Secretary of State for Environment. She is a Senior Lecturer in education at Lyon University and is the author of several books, including *Pas d'histoire, les femmes* and *Le ministère du possible.*

**Laurens Jan Brinkhorst** is Director-General for Environment, Consumer Protection and Nuclear Safety at the Commission of the European Communities, Brussels. He was the Dutch Secretary of State for Foreign Affairs from 1973 to 1977, Parliamentary Party Leader of the Democrats 66 Party in 1981, and Head of the EC delegation in Japan from 1982 to 1987.

**Dr Francisco Chavarria** is the Managing Director of the Scientific Foundation of the Spanish Association against Cancer and a practising physician in Madrid. He is Vice-President of the International Society for Research on Civilization Diseases and on Environment (SIRMCE); President of the Ibero-American Society for the Protection of Life, Health and Environment, and chairs the admission commission of the Spanish Society of Medical Writers.

**Professor Jose Manuel Rodriguez Delgado,** Academician of the Royal Academy of Doctors in Spain, was for thirty years a professor and research director in physiology and psychiatry at the Autonomous University Medical School in Madrid, and then at the Ramon y Cajal Centre. He is now the Director of the Centre for Neurobiological Studies and Director of Research at LBE Pharma, in Madrid. Professor Delgado is also a member of numerous societies and editorial boards in the fields of psychophysiology, neurobiology and biobehavioural sciences.

**Dr Jacques Douchamps** works at the Centre Hospitalier Universitaire de Montigny-le-Tilleul, Belgium, and is involved in research on the effects on man of new drugs (especially psychotropic drugs) in the Clinical Pharmacology Unit of the Université Libre de Bruxelles. Dr Douchamps' fields of special interest are cerebral mechanisms and their modelling.

**Professor Paul Duvigneaud** is the author of *La Synthèse Ecologique,* and is Honorary Professor at the Université Libre de Bruxelles, Belgium, where he taught botany, plant systematics, pedology and ecology. His research work was centered on ecosystemic ecology and biogeochemistry, and much of it was done in intertropical Africa. Professor Duvigneaud was a founder of the International Biological Programme (IBP) and is a past president of SCOPE, the Special Committee on Problems of the Environment, which was derived from IBP and the International Committee of Scientific Unions.

**Professor Jean-Paul Escande** is Head of Department and teaches medicine at the Cochin-Tarnier Hospital in Paris. His work is focused on three main themes: basic cancer research, adapting hospitals to the necessities of modern life, and developing patient care methods which are non-constraining for them and for society.

**Professor Hugh Freeman** is Honorary Professor at the University of Salford, United Kingdom. He is Editor of the British Journal of Psychiatry and a member of the Royal College of Psychiatrists.

**Professor Corneliu E. Giurgea** is Head of the Pharmacology Department at the Catholic University of Louvain-la-Neuve, Belgium. He is a scientific consultant to the Union Chimique Belge and the author of several books on psychopharmacology. Before 1969, he was Section Head of the Physiology Institute, Rumanian Academy.

**Professor Joseph Hautvast** teaches in the Department of Human Nutrition, Agricultural University of Wageningen, the Netherlands, where he directs an international postgraduate course in nutrition for students from developing countries. He is the Secretary-General of the International Union of Nutrition Sciences. Professor Hautvast's special areas of interest are the role of diet in cardiovascular diseases and cancer, children's growth and energy supply, and dietary trends of the future and their consequences for agriculture and health.

**Dr F.W. Häussler** works as an interior architect with the Studio for the Creation of Buildings and Space, in Reutlingen, FRG. His field of interest is the influence of the built environment on the psychological and physical quality of life.

**Mr René Huyghe,** of l'Académie Française, is a renowned expert on art. He is Honorary Professor at the Collège de France, Paris, where he specialises in the psychology of the visual arts. He is a curator of several museums, Director of the Musée Jacquemart-André in Paris, organiser of many major exhibitions, an editor of art magazines, collaborator on films about art, and the author of several books, including *Histoire de l'Art Contemporain, Le Dialogue avec le Visible,* and *Les Signes du Temps et l'Art Moderne* .

**Professor Robert Impens** teaches and does research on plant physiology and environmental stress at the Department of Plant Biology, Faculté des Sciences Agronomiques, in Gembloux, Belgium. His fields of interest are air pollution monitoring, waste recycling and urban forestry.

**Dr Marianne Klees** is a psychologist at the Queen Fabiola Children's Hospital in Brussels, Belgium, and teaches on learning disabilities in children and remedial techniques at the Faculty of Psychology and Pedagogy, Université Libre de Bruxelles.

**Professor Friedhelm Korte** is the Director of the Institute für ökologische Chimie at the Technical University of Munich, FRG, and President of the International Academy of Environmental Safety. His scientific interests are environmental chemistry, ecotoxicology and chemical carcinogenicity and mutagenicity. He is also a consultant to the World Health Organization and President of the Commission on Toxicology of IUPAC (International Union of Pure and Applied Chemistry).

**Dr Wilfried Kreisel** is Director of the Division of Environmental Health of the World Health Organization, Geneva. He joined WHO after having been Assistant Professor at the Institut für Umweltschutz und Planung at the University of Dortmund, FRG, and then working for nine years in Korea, Malaysia and the Philippines.

**Robert Krieps** has been Minister of Justice and Minister of Cultural Affairs as well as Minister of the Environment of the Grand Duchy of Luxembourg since 1984. A former president of the Luxembourg Socialist Party, he served as Minister of Education, of Justice, and of Cultural Affairs from 1974–79. In addition to practising law, Mr Krieps has also been a lecturer at the Universities of Nancy and Brussels.

**Dr Mohammed Mansour** is a research scientist specialising in the kinetics of photochemical and oxidation processes, at the Gesellschaft für Strahlen- und Umweltforschung (GSF) in Munich, FRG. In 1975 he joined the Institut für ökologische Chimie, which has as its main focus the development of test methods for ecotoxicological research and human health. Dr Mansour also has organised and directed a series of ecotoxicological studies for SIRMCE.

**Dr Federico Mayor** was appointed Director General of UNESCO in 1987, after having been Deputy Director General from 1978 to 1981. As a pharmacist and biochemist, he was successively Professor of Biochemistry at the Universities of Granada and Madrid, Director of the Severo Ochoa Molecular Biology Centre, and President of the Scientific and Technical Research Consultative Committee of the Spanish Government. He has been a member of the Spanish and European Parliaments, the Spanish Minister of Education and Science, and Director of the Institute of the Sciences of Man. Dr Mayor's book *Tomorrow is always too late,* is being translated into English.

**Professor Léopold Molle** is a member of the Royal Academy of Medicine of Belgium. Professor Emeritus at the Université Libre de Bruxelles since 1986, he has taught toxicology, drug analysis and cosmetology, and directed the Laboratories of Analytical Chemistry, Inorganic Pharmaceutical Chemistry, and Toxicology at the ULB Faculty of Medecine and Pharmacy. He is President and Director of the Central Laboratory of Toxicology in Brussels, Vice-President and member of the scientific council of SIRMCE, and a member of numerous scientific associations.

**Dr Antonius F.W. Morselt** is a cell biologist in the Faculty of Medicine at the University of Amsterdam. He has been working for the past nine years on the application of cell biology techniques to the detection of damage by environmental pollutants and his monograph on this subject is forthcoming. Dr Morselt is currently researching individual susceptibility to environmental pollutants, in cooperation with several researchers in the Netherlands as well as the National Institutes of Environmental Health of Japan and Finland.

**Professor Jean-Marie Pelt** teaches plant biology and pharmacognosis at the University of Metz, France. He is President of the European Institute of Ecology and of the European Foundation for Man, Nature and Life. Professor Pelt has written several books about plants, drugs and medicines, and has been involved in a number of television productions on plants and medicine.

**Peter Russell** is a British writer, lecturer, philosopher, and consultant. The author of *The Global Brain*, his fields of expertise are psychology and future studies.

**Dr Micheline Song** is Chargée de Cours at the Faculty of Medicine at the Université Libre de Bruxelles, Belgium, and is also Head of the Dermatology Clinic.

**Dr Emile Tockert** is a pediatrician and the Luxembourg representative of the International Physicians for the Prevention of Nuclear War, which was awarded the Nobel Peace Prize in 1985.

**Dr Mostafa K. Tolba** has been Executive Director of the United Nations Environment Programme (UNEP) since 1976 and holds the rank of Under-Secretary General of the United Nations. While Professor of Microbiology at the University of Cairo, Dr Tolba in 1965 joined the Egyptian Cabinet as Under-Secretary of State in the Ministry of Education, and from 1971 to 1973 was appointed Cabinet Minister of Youth and served as President of the Egyptian Academy of Scientific Research and Technology.

**Professor René C. Truhaut** has been Professor Emeritus of Toxicology at the Faculty of Pharmaceutical and Biological Sciences at the Université René Descartes since 1978, in Paris, where he had been the Director of the Teaching and Research Unit on the Action Mechanisms of Medicines and Toxics. For twenty-five years he was Professor of Toxicology at the Faculty of Pharmacy, Paris. He is the president of several international committees, and, until mid-1988, was Chairman of the Scientific Advisory Committee to Examine the Toxicity and Ecotoxicity of Chemical Compounds, of the European Commission.

**Dr Ing Wolfgang A.Volkrodt** was Director of Development in the field of electrical engineering for Siemens Corporation, where he was responsible for the application of new knowledge to new products. He has been an independent consultant since 1980.

**Dr Jeff G. Vos** is Director of Immunology and Head of the Laboratory for Pathology at the National Institute of Public Health and Environmental Protection, Bilthoven, The Netherlands. He received his Ph.D. from the University of Utrecht, where he studied the toxicology of polychlorinated biphenyls and their impurities. Co-authors with Dr Vos are H. Van Loveren and P.W. Wester, both of whom work at Bilthoven, and A.D. Vethaak, of the Tidal Water Division of the Public Works Department, Ministry of Transport and Public Works, the Netherlands.

**Paul Weber** is Assistant-Director of the Labour Inspectorate, Ministry of Labour, Luxembourg, and was formerly Head of the Division of International Affairs and Planning at the Ministry of Environment, Luxembourg. In 1981 and 1984, he presided over the Environment Group of the Council of the European Communities. In 1987/88 he was the official representative of the Ministry of Environment for all matters relating to the European Year of the Environment (EYE).

# Preface

This book is a concise summary of the international symposium **Man...Health...Environment,** which was hosted by the Luxembourg Government 3–5 March 1988, as one of the major closing events of the European Year of the Environment.

The aim of the conference was to bring together international experts to consider the environment crisis from a technical/symptomatic point of view as well as from a more philosophical/holistic perspective – to expose the relationship between human activity and problems of environment and health.

An unexpected consensus seemed to run through the whole meeting, a refrain as it were, which I would like to summarise thus:

> Short-sightedness and fragmented thinking has led us to decisions which disturbed the balance in nature. The undesired fall-out has harmed the ecology and our own health. While we must continue to seek practical solutions for repairing the damage caused to our environment, we must also look at *ourselves* and seek means for broadening our understanding and sensitivity in order to avoid catastrophes in the future.

Towards the end of the meeting, a clear call came for a new spirituality, a rediscovering of the deeper human values. An ethical system should be put into practice which is based on our accumulated experience rather than mere ideological dogma. Such an ethical approach should include ecological, social and both psychological and physical health considerations.

It is obvious that the fundamental shift in our thinking which is necessary to bring human society and the environment back to balance cannot be achieved through conferences alone. What we face is a problem of education.

Unless education, whether at home or at school, plants the seeds for a broad and integrated understanding of ourselves and nature, a long-term solution to environmental *and* health problems does not seem possible.

Einstein and other great scientists have forewarned us that although the great scientific discoveries and their application through technology have completely changed the world we live in, they have not changed our thinking, and that unless we radically change our thinking – and perhaps even our whole approach to life – our collective survival is at stake.

It is not too late to meet this great challenge which humanity has brought upon itself. At least the tone of the Luxembourg meeting suggested this: it was a tone of hope and optimism.

*Robert Krieps,*
*Minister of the Environment*
*Luxembourg*

# Introduction

by Professor Léopold Molle

Our society seems to be at a major crossroads. Ages ago, with our marvellous brains and wondrously flexible thumbs, we set in motion a wheel of technology that has now gathered great speed. The revolutions of this wheel have brought enormous benefits to the industrialized societies: the ability to grow food in great abundance; medicines that prevent and cure diseases; improved hygiene to promote better health; a comfortable interior climate whatever the weather; networks of transportation and communication which reduce distances, favouring more and closer human contact and increasing commercial development; and a material wealth which is more equal and universal than it has ever been before. And the wheel is not stopping. It gathers ever greater speed as our inventions and technological applications become more and more sophisticated.

But the wheel has also brought chaos and destruction: polluted rivers, seas and air, dying forests, contaminated food, a depleted ozone layer, and the threat from nuclear weapons and disasters. We are now realising that along with health protection our technological revolution has also given us a host of 'civilization diseases': cancer, heart diseases, psychological disorders, high blood pressure, depression of the immune system, and other health risks caused by chemical and physical pollution. Not only have we damaged our environment, but we have endangered our human minds and bodies.

While we in the industrialized world begin to grapple with this realisation, developing nations are – rightfully – seeking the benefits of the wheel. But we do not know how to pass on the benefits without the dangers, so they too are experiencing the bad with the good – desertification, destruction of the rain forests, exhaustion of natural resources. Our whole globe is endangered; life and nature as we know it is threatened.

Yet we cannot blame man, because he is inherently a 'sorcerer's apprentice'. It is the very nature of man that moves him to try to survive, to master the elements and adapt his environment. Still, the danger we are facing today comes from the profound mutation that our environment is undergoing. Thus it is not sufficient for man to possess 'savoir faire' or know-how; he must also have 'savoir consommer' or 'know-how-to-use'.

So we are at a crossroads. We must choose a direction. Will we continue hurtling towards unconscious destruction of our environment – and thus of ourselves? Or will we try to turn onto another path where we can undo the damage we have done and learn to steer the wheel safely?

This book represents a meeting of minds on these issues. It brings together the thoughts and feelings of highly respected men and women from different parts of Europe who are specialists in a wide diversity of fields: ecotoxicology, immunology, medicine, nutrition, biochemistry, physics, psychiatry, education, politics, international government, architecture, the fine arts, and philosophy. Not only do these writers represent different national cultures and different disciplines, but they also speak with the voices of three different generations.

What are they telling us? The scientists try to explain the ecosystem and its interrelationships, and relate how the science of ecotoxicology was born. They trace the development of the environmental crisis, point out the linkages, and identify the damage that has been recognised. Then they show us how, aided by precise tools created with modern technology, the environmental sciences are beginning to invent ways to assess risks to nature and to human health before action is taken: before chemicals are manufactured and transported, before pesticides are sold and applied, before medicines and food additives are prescribed and imbibed.

The researchers in the medical sciences pinpoint the injuries to man's body and mind from misuse of and damage to our environment. Their contributions show us how medicine is moving away from a rather arbitrary division between physical and emotional factors and is increasingly taking a whole view of the human being. Moreover, in some fields of medicine – such as geriatrics, nutrition, psychiatry, etc. – people are being seen holistically: as individuals, as members of their community, and as part of their social and physical environment.

The architects and urban planners represented in this book tell us about their research, their experiments, and the way their designs have incorporated lessons from the natural and human sciences. These papers point to the gains acquired by learning from the natural environment and warn of the consequences of not adapting the man-made environment to peoples' basic natural needs.

Our quality of life is inextricably linked to the environment, say the politicians and the representatives of international organisations. They think and speak in international terms because their day-to-day work has taught them that the environment knows no frontiers. These are the people who constantly face the demands of competing public interests pulling in different directions. They are elected and appointed to find a way to combine economic prosperity and technical progress with an improved quality of life, but there are no magic wands provided with each office. So, as they explain here, theirs is the art of the possible with struggles such as the World Health Organization's fight to provide the world's population with safe drinking water, UNEP's historic Montreal Protocol to protect the ozone layer, the European Community's battles to get the EC's environmental directives implemented by its member states. Those in national and international posts dealing with the environment constantly face the dilemma of seeking decisions that strike a balance between the need to impose human projects on the natural environment and the need to preserve the richness and integrity of that environment.

To the philosphers and artists, our society seems lopsided. The human scale of values has become unbalanced and weighed down by an undue emphasis on efficiency, material benefits, over-concentration on logic and rationality, an explosion of factual information. We are hurrying headlong, but where? There is a sense of distress and insecurity in our society, an oppressive awareness of entropy – that the universe is gradually, inevitably running down.

We must heed these signals. It is time to steer science towards creative caring – to use the environmental sciences to restore our equilibrium within nature and guide our future endeavours towards creating a more fulfilling material and spiritual environment.

We have not paid enough attention to the development of our ethical, emotional and spiritual intelligence – to our innate senses of values. The philosophers and artists believe this is the force which must steer humankind's technological wheel. But in most of us it lies dormant. Thus we each must take the time to reflect, to recognise these values, so that our behaviour as individuals and as a society can reflect a true balance between the rational on one side and the ethical, emotional and spiritual on the other.

For some time, say the scientists, politicians, artists and philosophers, the rational has weighed too heavily in the scales. It is now time to go back to balance.

Chapter 1

# The spirit of René Dubos, or the dangers of a fragmentary approach to ecology[1]

by Jean-Paul Escande

The French philosopher Blaise Pascal, in his *Pensées,* wrote: 'The heart has its reasons that reason knows not. We see it in all things'. With this in mind, ecologists can be divided up into ecologists of the heart and ecologists of reason.

## *Ecologists of the heart*

The ability to symbolise is one of the essential characteristics of the human mind. Every day, every hour, every minute and in all circumstances human beings symbolise. A play, a story, the birth of a concept creates an emotion

---

1 René Dubos was a micro-biologist, experimental pathologist and scientific humanist. He lived exactly eighty-one years, from 20 February 1901 to 20 February 1982. Trained as an agronomist, he left his native France at the age of twenty-one for Rome and then the USA. From 1927 to his death, he worked at the Rockefeller Institute, later to become Rockefeller University. As a researcher and thinker, he had a profound influence on his time, laying the groundwork for the discovery of antibiotics (1927–39), defining the modern concept of health, particularly in *Mirage of Health* (1960–70), and creating an original, working concept of environment (1970–82). His books include *Man, Medicine and Environment*, *So Human an Animal*, *Reason Awake: Science for Man*, and *A God Within.*

in us. A hazy and vague cloud settles and crystallises on that which spawned it. This starting point becomes a symbol. None of us can escape this function and it is rightly said to be distinctive to human beings.

Many ecologists, listening to their hearts, let their emotional reactions take priority. Words like 'nuclear', 'chemical', 'natural' or even 'vaccine' have become emotionally highly charged and lead many of us to believe that we are assuming rights which run counter to the natural order of things.

In what follows I shall judge no one. But I hope to show that emotional reactions often reflect not only the recognition of a blow against the natural order but also a particular conditioning of the mind.

People's emotional reactions can, for example, be quite different depending on the environment they inhabit. Small groups opposed to vaccination or antibiotics on ecological grounds exist in rich, industrialised countries – not in less favoured countries where disease spells disaster and where vaccines or the most chemical of medicines remain a privilege for the most fortunate. Still reflecting on the conditioning of the human mind, what would have happened if Louis Pasteur's discoveries had been used in a horrible bacteriological war and if nuclear power had been confined to energy production and had never interested the military? Would we not see today powerful movements organised to stop the construction of great bacteriological laboratories while nuclear power stations would be built in total indifference?

Taking the opposite view, it must be said that very often emotional reactions express a feeling against which we must not fight, for emotions are often right when they oppose the wild pretensions of egotistical people concerned only with their desire for personal gain or individual power. Ecology of the heart by itself is weak. But if it can be applied in a society which can take account of emotional factors, it is an essential force. And any society which cannot incorporate basic emotional values into what it builds will slowly dry up and die.

## *Ecologists of reason*

The nature of the human brain enables us to perceive the world other than through our emotions. And because we can see it this other way we can take it apart and see its springs and joints. This is the field of science.

For a long time human ecology was an offshoot of sociology. In 1939, for a book entitled *An outline of the principles of sociology*, A.B. Hollingshead wrote an important chapter called precisely 'Human ecology'. It was not until the early 1960s that scientists, and biologists in particular, applied themselves to the study of ecology. The role of René Dubos in this was exemplary and decisive.

I shall try to explain this changeover. After Avery had shown that hereditary characteristics were passed on by a single molecule, DNA, and Crick and Watson had discovered its double helix structure which carried the genetic code, an enormous amount of interest began to develop among biologists in the study of the secrets of life through chemistry. The idea of 'the force of life' had a hard time fitting into this new and purely material way of thinking. Molecular biology had thrown life out of its studies. Because they were concerned with its mystery, ecological biologists picked it up. For them life was not only a replication of nucleic acid and a body of proteic synthesis completed here and there by a few mutations. It was not only the use of chemical energy to synthesise and transform organic matter. For them life was a creative process shaping order out of the disorder of matter and tirelessly engendering new or even unforeseen structures and properties by making combinations which qualititively transcend their constituent parts. On this a biological ecology could be built which sought to make an inventory of the effects of human activity on nature, people and human health.

Yet the very nature of science forces us to consider problems one by one, and scientific ecology has sometimes lost sight of the whole picture of the problems facing it. This tendency has continued to grow. Much of the work on problems as serious as the depletion of the ozone layer, marine pollution, acid rain, the dangers of radioactivity and deforestation is often too easily satisfied with measuring the phenomenon without seeing the real significance of the measurement taken. Einstein said that science allowed us to measure anything, but that the measurements we obtained were often useless. In ecology, perhaps more so than in any other discipline, we should not forget his words.

Fragmentary ecological studies, which flatter themselves on setting seriousness and precision against the vagueness of uncontrolled emotional reactions, are often more concerned with dramatic problems than with the successes of human enterprise. They study the disastrous effects of oil slicks more readily than the successes of those who through effort, imagination and practical work succeed in improving coastlines. It is true that there are meetings to celebrate the beauty of a site where nature has been preserved. But most scientists would feel they were not being really 'scientific' if they put forward a project to a scientific organisation to carry out work on the beauty of a site or its characteristically gentle way of life. This self-censorship is becoming a handicap, because science, anxious to contribute to people's happiness, has not only the duty to give them technical devices which encourage their natural tendencies to do as little as possible.; it must also analyse scientifically all the examples of environmental success which contribute to human happiness. There are many such examples. Can we not then avoid an excessive and harmful fragmentation of scientific research and leave the dark, negative paths for the lighted paths of positive thinking. I think this is possible, and to prove it I shall start with a story which is old, but not well known – the origins of the 1972 United Nations Conference on the Human Environment – afterwards known as the Stockholm Conference.

## The spirit of 'Stockholm 1972'

The Stockholm Conference was such a success and it has become so commonplace to applaude it that to come back to it now might seem superfluous. But the origins of the conference and the spirit which fired it are worth relating.

It is said that in the early 1960s René Dubos had chosen to defend the then somewhat unacceptable idea that the scientific community should not leave the study of ecology to sociologists alone. Ecology seemed to him to be the life science par excellence. But this approach did not meet with unanimity, either among the scientific community or even at Rockefeller University, where he worked, because biologists saw ecology as a land full of pools of quicksand. By 1971, however, his ideas had gained a considerable amount of ground, and René Dubos was asked to head the group of experts preparing the Stockholm Conference. The circumstances which led to his being asked are of great interest. In his letter to Dubos, Maurice Strong, the Conference's Secretary General, said this: 'This letter is to commission you formally to establish and serve as chairman of an international group of experts to prepare a report on the state of the world environment. ... The main purpose of this report is to help establish a conceptual frame of reference for the work of the conference on specific substantive problems.' In fact when Dubos was designated, the group of experts had already done a considerable amount of work under the direction of Barbara Ward and the report was nearly ready, but it seemed satisfactory neither to Ward nor Strong.

On 13 July 1971, after reading the report, Dubos wrote a few rather detached remarks and a few criticisms. He seemed interested but no more than that. 'Dear Barbara, Quel tour de force! Repeatedly, I feared that your intense interest – so excitingly obvious – in the history of the cosmos and of life on earth would make you forget that the Stockholm Conference had more prosaic concerns. But in each case you brought the reader back – naturally – to practical issues and thus made natural history directly relevant to environmental problems.' Then followed a few detailed points on the report. Perhaps his attitude was explained by the postscript: 'These notes written in bed as I am to enter New York hospital. Have lost 12 pounds during the past four weeks, which may be a good way of starting post-retirement life'.

However, on 28 September, he had recovered and wrote Barbara Ward a letter which conveyed his optimistic vision in spite of all.

> Dear Barbara, I had hesitated writing you with suggestions concerning the book, because I know how difficult it is to change a structure after it has begun to develop its own genius. But Mr Brian Johnson, with whom I spent a most rewarding hour last week, assures me that the ideas I had in mind are quite congenial to you and would reinforce your own attitude. In brief, I believe that:
> a) being human implies managing nature. I like to use the word 'stewardship' precisely because it is somewhat ambiguous: man acts as a steward either for a higher order of things, or for mankind as an entity.
> b) the history of the European land, and of several parts of Asia, shows that man can create out of wilderness new environments which are ecologically sound, economically profitable, and esthetically rewarding.
> c) nature is so resilient that it can be restored to a condition of quality if man provides help and guidance. From what I have heard, the cost may not be as exorbitant – per capita – as usually believed. ... I wish that a serious attempt be made to develop *social* accounting for a few specific cases of social recovery.
> d) implicit in my attitude is a kind of faith in man ( ... the evidence of things unseen!). Wherever free men are involved, trend is not destiny.

René Dubos gave Barbara Ward the boost she needed. On this new basis, the report doubled in size. To each chapter was added a section dealing with activities of human creativity – positive actions in the ecological movement bringing together emotional values and purely technical data. By putting together pure science, social science and emotional response, Stockholm was the success we now know it to have been.

## The 'Five Es'

The spirit of Stockholm brought to light perhaps the major problem facing humanity: how to pose problems without neglecting any of their dimensions.

Since the seventeenth century, since Descartes and Bacon, we have been able to solve problems posed in scientific terms by scientific methods. But what we normally cannot do, or can no longer do, is to pose human problems in terms which leave room for human realities not measureable in exact terms. We have witnessed the triumph of the motto of the Chicago World's Fair: 'Science discovers, industry applies, man conforms'. But in fact man refuses to conform. We need balance, discovery, creation and emotion; the need for a general theory of ecology tending towards the attainment of positive objectives would seem an absolute priority.

It is time then to draw attention to a theory put forward by René Dubos a short time before his death, the theory of the 'Five Es': Ecosystem – Economy – Energy – Esthetics – Ethics.

The Five E theory postulates that applications of scientific discoveries are only valuable if they can combine with the emotional basis of human life, and *a contrario* those people who are the most prone to emotional response have a duty to think seriously about the beneficial repercussions of scientific discoveries before getting carried away and raising their voices against them. A science-emotion dialectic therefore underlies the whole Five E theory.

## *Ecosystem*

Everywhere people settle, a deep conflict arises between them and nature. Dreaming of lost paradises, certain people have always believed that conflict was not inevitable. So throughout human history, two opposing tendencies must always have been set face to face. Cro-Magnon men and women probably argued amongst themselves about the utility of cutting down certain trees, killing certain animals or leaving here or there the residues of their human activities. Saint Francis of Assisi was a model for nature preservationists who wanted to blend with nature without modifying anything. But the Benedictine monks offered a model which was much nearer to what a majority of people think of as man's duty to the earth. By cutting down forests, planting crops, draining swamps and raising magnificent buildings, the Benedictines believed they were following the path of divine creation rather than inflicting wounds on the local ecosystem.

In fact, the opposition between preservationists and interventionists is less sharp than it would appear. For what preservationists call nature is in fact often far removed from 'original' nature. Our 'countryside' is not wild but humanised. We are so used to gazing on and marvelling at open spaces, groves and forests, well-drained streams and rivers, that we tend to forget that all this was created by human beings. Nature before the neolithic period bore no comparison to that which has existed since man intervened. With the exception of the polar regions, mountain tops and deserts, practically all of nature in Europe has been humanised. And it is this humanised nature we want to protect. Science and technology now enable us to give this protection, and to plan it on solid foundations. They allow us to envisage the conservation of the planet's resilience and power of self-recovery anywhere – on land and in the sea. But the preservation of localised ecosystems – biotopes – involves great human vigilance with respect to the other 4 Es.

### *Economy*

The definition of economy I propose to adopt in an ecological perspective is the second one in the Concise Oxford Dictionary: 'careful use of resources'. A country's economy must contribute to 'carefully using' the abilities acquired by people through scientific discoveries and cultural and technical creation. Unfortunately economics (and economists) is still at the stage biology was at before Pasteur, Darwin or Ehrlich. Periodic stock market collapses, monetary confusion and the inability of the richest to respect and contribute to the development of the poorest not only show up greed, rapaciousness and egotism, but prove that economics is a discipline still in its infancy. Economics can only partially fulfill its task because it does not want to satisfy that emotional part of human beings we call the soul.

What economist would not burst out laughing if he were asked to incorporate into his figures the absolute necessity of letting the inhabitants of major industrial cities contemplate the stars shining in the firmament? None. And yet, at night in the country, that same economist, raising his head and seeing a shooting star, perceives himself immediately as part of the whole cosmos. And at that moment he feels neither ridiculous nor crazy. And he is right not to feel so! He ought perhaps to take that into account when he drafts notes or compiles dossiers, or when he is in board meetings.

### *Energy*

The economy and energy consumption are closely linked. Energy production is the *sine qua non* of the development of industrial economies. However, the deployment of massive quantities of energy poses ecological problems of the same scale. Landscapes ruined by mining, oil slicks, smoke pollution, nuclear waste – these anger us, make us ill or even kill us.

Economists often refuse to hear or see what is going on and even cleverly justify themselves by attacking the exaggerated claims of those who give in to extreme emotional reactions. This is how the debate over nuclear power has become clouded. It is true that nuclear energy certainly presents dangers. But the accident at Chernobyl must not make us forget the countless deaths due to the mining of coal and the extraction of oil. Fundamentalist ecologists should in fact, when going past a nuclear power station, be delighted as they contemplate one of their finest victories.

According to the rules, attention has been paid to the architecture, the surrounding land is cultivated, streams and rivers are well kept and safety measures to avoid accidents are far superior to those in other sectors of industrial activity. In France the nuclear industry holds the record for the lowest number of industrial accidents, far lower than in the clothing industry, for example. There is a lesson to be learnt here.

In the relationship between ecology and energy, we must not pursue battles we have already won, but concentrate on those areas where everything or nearly everything remains to be done. Oil tankers flushing out their holds at sea, acid rain, smog, or the blackened buildings of cities, are examples of the work remaining to be done to solve problems associated with energy.

## *Esthetics*

We often tend to look on the need for esthetics as frivolous or capricious. And yet, after our need for water and food, followed by putting a suitable temperature around our bodies whatever the climate or season, esthetics is perhaps our next need. Cultures and fashions may vary, certainly, but harmony of form and subtle matching of colours and sounds are genuine human needs. So ecology must, and does, concern itself with esthetics. Keeping birds alive requires ethics, but a silent spring, with no birds singing in the air or in the trees, would hurt our esthetic sense. The rubbish piled up in too many streets of too many cities, urban decay and dirt, horizons blotted out by lugubrious high rise buildings, the leprous growth of flaking paint on walls – all this shocks our visual esthetics.

Esthetics, finally, is about all our senses, and ecology must ultimately be able to pride itself on inventing a type of man-nature relationship which can satisfy all these senses.

## *Ethics*

Ecological ethics asks the question about the duties of people towards the rest of creation: other people, animals, plants, the earth's crust. Human beings have, to a certain extent, been split off from the rest because of their brains, which have given them an ability to discover, create and symbolise. So, freed from pure biological determinism and endowed in any given situation not with a wide-ranging free will, but with a restricted choice of proposals put to them by their imaginations, human beings can – responsibly – choose the path to take: of beauty, Good and goodness, or of ugliness, Evil and badness.

## Out of Nature

We have two choices before us. The first is to submit to those restrictive scientific and technological forces we ourselves – latter-day Frankensteins – have created, and whose productions we too often take for exactitude and truth. A future based on such 'truth' is a mirage.

The second is for ecologists to change the direction of human activity by asking constantly every entrepreneur, builder and researcher: 'What does this project need so that all Five Es are met?'

René Dubos liked to use the ambiguous expression 'out of nature' to describe the place of man in the order of things. We came out of nature and are hence part of it, but we are also outside it. It is this which is both our specificity and the great cause of human ecology. This cause can be won if in all human enterprise we try to strike a balance between the Five Es – Ecosystem, Economy, Energy, Esthetics and Ethics.

# Part I

# The Scientists

Chapter 2

# Ecology and man: biosphere, noosphere, sophiosphere

by Paul Duvigneaud

Man has been practising ecology for ages, without realising it, in order to survive. Ecology is the study of relationships between living beings and their non-living environment. It turned into a science around the end of the 19th century, with the works of Haekel and Reiter. Classical ecology studies nature and the results of human activity on it.

There is much concern nowadays about the evolution of the world, and it is being realised more and more that our planet functions as one big ecosystem, of which man is a vital component. This means that human activity may direct the trends of the planetary evolution, but that we are nevertheless submitted, like other living beings, to the general laws which control the functioning of an ecosystem – the laws of nature.

But what is an ecosystem? For non-ecologists it may be useful to summarise here a few general notions and to define a few common terms as they are used for plant communities, before attempting to extend the ecological approach to man.

## General notions

Environmental factors (light, heat, water, mineral and organic substrates) determine *biotopes*, where living organisms of various kinds and numbers meet to form *biosystems* (mixtures of populations belonging to different species).

The plants, animals and micro-organisms in a biosystem develop associative links and form communities or *biocenoses*. For modern ecology, the integration of biocenoses to their environmental factors into functional *ecosystems*, where they are influenced by their environment and influence it themselves, is essential for the maintenance of life on earth. This is the holistic or holocoenotic concept.

Plants and animals – and thus biocenoses – become metamorphosed, i.e. change their physiognomy under the influence of the environment. A biocenosis such as a forest exists in different *formations* according to its environment, e.g. temperate deciduous forest, or mediterranean evergreen hard-leafed forest, or conifer boreal forest, etc.

Plant formations progress dynamically through a *succession* of pioneer and intermediate stages to a *climax*, which is a formation in a stationary equilibrium with the climate of the time. The climax may regress, due to natural or man-made disturbances; in forest clearings made by fire, storms or parasites, the succession starts again from square one. A *biome* is a climax botanogeocenosis, including all the animals and micro-organisms within it.

In the modern world, man is an important component of many types of ecosystems. The *Essay of an ecology of man* by M. Sorre (1947) shows the diversity and complexity of the human influence on nature – an influence well classified by Ellenberg (1984) in his study of the ways farms have been built in Western Europe.

## Functioning of a natural ecosystem

A natural ecosystem is structured in space and in time. It involves a trophic network (who eats what) starting with producer plants (producing a biomass by photosynthesis or chemiosynthesis), followed by consumers (herbivorous, carnivorous of several orders, parasites, scavengers), decomposers, mineralizers and symbionts (nitrogen-fixing organisms, mycorrhizes). In order to function, the ecosystem needs energy, water and some minerals essential to life. The study of the cycles and balances of these elements is important in ecological work.

### *Energy*

The source of energy is mainly solar radiation, in a wide range of wavelengths expressed in microns (μ). It includes:

- bactericide, long wavelength UV rays (0.29 to 0.38 μ): the more toxic and energetic UV rays are stopped above 25 km by an ozone layer;
- visible light (0.38 to 0.78 μ): for photosynthesis, plants absorb mainly the purple-blue and orange-red radiation;
- near (or short) infra-red rays (0.78 to 3.0 μ): their role in the functioning of ecosystems is minor;
- far or long infra-red rays (3.0 to 100 μ), also called thermal radiation, which have a high calorific effect.

Thirteen per cent of the total solar radiation is captured by steam, carbon dioxide and dust, and transformed in the atmosphere into long infra-red rays. Another part of the radiation is reflected on the surface of the earth: the *albedo*. The albedo percentage is highest for the short infra-red and for yellow and green light (the colours least absorbed by plants). For thermal radiation, the albedo coefficient is about four per cent for vegetation or water, but eleven per cent for bare sand.

Some radiation is absorbed by the biocenoses and some by the ground: both are largely converted into thermal energy. Heat has to be re-radiated back into space to avoid a continuous warming of the system, incompatible with life. Warm air moves up into the atmosphere by convection; its replacement by cold air is the origin of winds (eolian energy, also available to ecosystems). Other ways of dissipating heat are evaporation from water surfaces or plant transpiration. The condensation of water vapour as rain is directly related to the extent of this evapotranspiration. Hence the vital role of forests in rain patterns.

## *Water*

There is usually a balance drawn between water import – rain, snow, fog – and water export by evapotranspiration, surface flow, ground infiltration feeding the water table, and finally the flow into rivers.

Water circulation in ecosystems, both terrestrial and aquatic, gives organisms the water they need and brings about cycles and fluxes of mineral and organic nutrients – sap circulation, leaching of leaves by rain, etc.

## *Mineral nutrients*

Mineral nutrients are distributed in the soil, the water, the air, and in the biomass of the biocenosis. They are circulated with the sap during the year, from root *absorption* in the soil to the various organs of the plants where they are *retained*; they also move along the food chains. The mineral nutrients are then *restituted* to the soil by leaching, the fall of dead matter and the action of the decomposers/remineralisers.

In addition to this internal cyclic pattern (absorption = retention + restitution), the ecosystem imports nutrients, as well as some toxic elements – lead, cadmium, copper etc. – , from the rock-bed or the atmosphere. Some imports are exported again by draining into rivers, lakes and sea, or by wind erosion. Gaseous compounds, such as ammonia or hydrogen sulphide volatilise as a result of bacterial action in the fermenting organic debris on the soil. In a stationary, balanced ecosystem, exports are approximately equal to imports.

### *Productivity and biomass*

The functioning of the ecosystem results in the production of a certain amount of *biomass* (dry weight of organic matter); the rate of production of biomass, by hectare per year for instance, is the *productivity*. (See Figure 2.1.)

## Ecosystem dynamics: reactions to stress due to natural or man-made disturbances

In nature, an ecosystem can be submitted to energy-linked disturbances – storms, fires, droughts, abnormal cold, etc. – liable to modify its development. What is a detrimental stress at one level of the ecosystem can be beneficial at another: for example, periodic fire in a steppe or a mediterranean forest is a stress for many organisms which will be injured or killed, but not for the ecosystem which is adapted to fire and could not persist without it.

Natural stress is mainly acute, i.e. periodical, and ecosystems have adapted themselves to it either by a high resistance, or through *redundancy* (replacement of sensitive species by better adapted ones), or by a resilience which allows them to reconstruct themselves in a short time.

In industrial society, man-made stress, on the contrary, is often chronic, i.e. continuous, and linked to a chemical pollution unknown in the original ecosystem. Ecosystems under stress show a tendency to modify their normal functioning: respiration increases, thus productivity decreases, and geochemical fluxes increase while biological cycles are hampered.

Depending on the level of pollution, the ecosystem passes through a series of damage stages, from insignificant to collapse, resulting in the definitive loss of its self-repair potential.

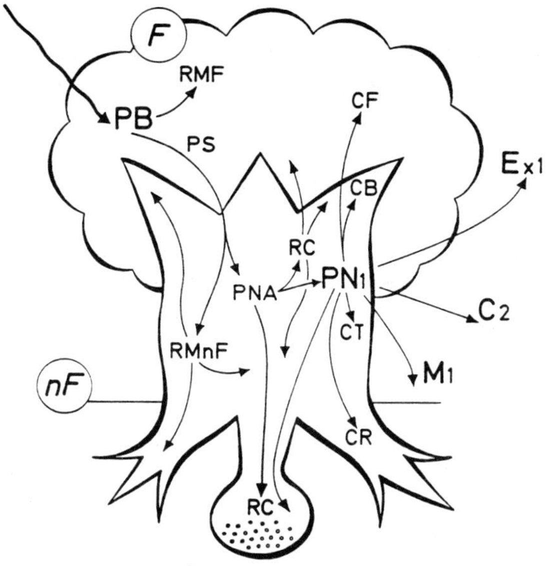


Figure 2.1 Energy fluxes and production of organic matter

From the upper left: leaves of green plants (F) using photosynthesis, convert $CO_2$ from the air and water from the ground into organic assimilates (glucides) and oxygen. PB is the raw productivity (quantity of assimilates per hectare/per year). Some of the assimilates (RMF) are 'burnt' (by respiration, with release of $CO_2$) to provide energy to maintain the leaf system F. The surplus (PS) provides energy to maintain nF, the non-photosynthetic part of the system, (branches, stems, roots). What is left (RC) is used for the construction of new leaves, flowers, fruits and seeds (CF), new branches (CB), stems (CT), roots (CR), and for the storage of reserve materials. The total of the materials produced (biomass) in one year on one hectare of the biocenosis is the net primary productivity (PN1).

Ex1 represents the part of the biomass exported by wind or rain (leaves, pollen, seeds, volatile resins).

C2 is the part consumed by predators (herbivorous, granivorous, etc.).

M1 represents dead matter, either attached to the tree (bark, dead wood) or falling on the ground (leaves, twigs, inflorescences, fruit, etc.). A large quantity of thin roots is also discarded on the ground.

The total increase of the biomass, after eliminating the losses in Ex1 and C2, is made up of increments in phytomass and in zoomass. Adding to it the increases in litter and humus (necromass) gives the net productivity of the biocenosis (PNB). A yearly organomass balance may be obtained by subtracting from PNB the necromasses produced during previous years.

## Hierarchy within ecosystems: ecolandscapes, ecoregions, biosphere

Within their environment, populations are part, in time and space, of various loosely defined groups: for example a forest biogeocenosis is made up of intricate ecosociologic groups, composed of bioindicators of light, temperature, humidity, soil, fertility, etc. A mosaïc of such forest biogeocenoses makes a forest landscape. Forests, fields and meadows make rural geolandscapes; urban and industrial areas form very complex ecolandscapes. A mosaïc of geo- and ecolandscapes forms an ecoregion, and the sum of the ecoregions, continental and oceanic, is the planet-sized *biosphere*, according to the Russian geochemist, W. Vernadsky, considered by many as the father of modern ecology (Vernadsky, 1924).

Landscape ecology should aim to create balanced rural landscapes – silva on hilltops, saltus on the slopes, and ager in the valleys – to prevent the impoverishment of hilltops, the erosion of slopes and the flooding of valleys, and to encourage beneficial water and nutrient balances. When a system of cultural, agricultural and industrial traditions, with favorable economic and social factors, corresponds to a balanced ecolandscape, the correct functioning of the ecoregion can then be called *ecodevelopment*.

## Taking man into account in the biosphere: the noosphere

The biosphere was studied in depth by Vernadsky in 1924-29. His works are a remarkable synthesis of what was known then in natural sciences, as seen from the angle of materialistic philosophy.

For him, life is the mightiest geological force on earth. It acts both chemically – metabolism of living beings – and mechanically – bed-rock decomposers, mixers, borers, transporters, etc. It involves the formation, at the surface of the mineral sphere, of a complex geological layer made up of biogenic materials , i.e. produced by life processes:

- living matter (no more than 1 per cent of the whole)
- dead matter of biological origin: either mineral (soil skeletons, loams, clays and their exchangeable ions) or organic (vegetable or animal litter, humus, peat).

During geological periods, living beings evolve and change, and the sequence of successive biospheres forms the metabiosphere. Taphological processes[1] have preserved remains of bygone biospheres for us to see (Lapo,

[1] Taphology is the study of the transformation of dead bodies into fossils.

1987). Fossilization transforms some biogenic substances into oil, coal, brown coal, or natural gas, which are our main energy sources.

About three million years ago, human beings appeared in the biosphere, at first just another natural element, as hunters/gatherers. But their influence on nature increased, thanks to fire and tools and the many effects of the domestication of animals. From about 60,000 years ago, as Homo sapiens, man applied his mind and ever-increasing knowledge to transform the natural biosphere even more (agriculture, industrialization, urbanisation). In this way, human beings have now become the mightiest geological force on the planet (Vernadsky, 1945): the discoveries of the human mind (noos in Greek ) applied to the well-being of humankind have transformed the biosphere into the noosphere.

In the 1920s, the mathematician and philosopher E. Le Roy and the paleontologist P. Teilhard de Chardin also used the concept of noosphere, but with a much more spiritualistic or even religious meaning – a kind of atmosphere of thought, spread around and above the biosphere.

The noosphere according to Vernadsky includes the agrosphere – cultivated areas, meadows, parks and gardens, paths and drives, hot-houses, fish ponds, etc. – and the technosphere – built-up areas, factories and workshops, airports, roads, etc.

Dansereau proposed a rational classification for the noosphere and for what is left of the biosphere. The categories take into account the escalation of man's hold over his environment. Areas can be:

- indigenous: pristine, unadulterated nature;
- colligenous: gathering, hunting and fishing;
- agrigenous: agriculture and sylviculture;
- fabrigenous: mining, manufacturing, production of energy;
- urbigenous: residence, trade, services, with a variable amount of greenery;
- cybernigenous: transport, administration, communication, monitoring activities, etc.

## *The productivity of the noosphere: carrying capacity and cultural capacity*

Considering the present noosphere (including the few parts of the biosphere which remain intact in inaccessible places) as a gigantic ecosystem, it is possible, knowing the relative areas of the different biomes and their biomass and productivity, to calculate the total biomass and productivity of the noosphere. This productivity, of about 150 billion tonnes of organic matter, could theoretically feed 160 billion vegetarian humans, or 40 billion humans on a mixed diet. This represents the *carrying capacity of the system,* allowing for mere survival (about 1200 kcal/man/day). But every person is entitled to a good life: we need more matter and energy to dress, to stay healthy, to have a comfortable home, to keep warm and to cook our food, to move around, to have leisure activities. Here we have to evaluate the *cultural capacity*, measured in kg of coal equivalent spent per capita per annum (Hardin, 1986): its world average is about fifty-nine times that of the present-day Ethiopian. (For the US citizen the average is more than three hundred times that of the Ethiopian.) If we admit that every citizen in the world is entitled to 'a good life', we must recognise that our estimate of the possible number of these citizens is much too high.

## Cities: the ecosystem urbs

A city is the most important and characteristic humanised ecosystem, and the best illustration of the noosphere. In contrast with 'sylva', the forest ecosystem, 'urbs' implies a concentration of human populations, and of fabrigenous, urbigenous and cybernigenous activities. It is the centre of a real anthropocenosis, into which all individuals bring their particular qualities as Homo biologicus, mentalis, socialis, economicus and nowadays circulans and intoxicatus.

### *The peculiarities of the urban ecosystem*

The urban ecosystem is distinguished from natural, semi-natural or agricultural ecosystems (silva, saltus, ager) by many fundamental characteristics: solar energy and rain water are replaced to a large extent by importations of electrical energy, of fossil fuels, and of piped water from distant sources. Human and animal food is also largely imported from the outside.

Instead of being wisely recycled, huge amounts of minerals are discarded in the gutter, as industrial or domestic smoke, and by waste-disposal. After they have polluted the water, the soil and the atmosphere of the city itself, they pollute and eutrophize the rivers and the ocean ('refuse ecosystem').

The urban ecosystem has some climatic characteristics of its own. The heat liberated by burning fossil fuels (in industry, domestic heating, cars, etc.) increases the temperature of the air and is responsible for the warmer 'thermal dome', of which the top lies above cities and industrial centres, while the fringe reaches the peripheral, greenery-studded sub-systems where the temperature is lower. On the other hand, the presence of a dome of dust and gaseous suspensions on large cities reduces the penetration of the sun's rays and contributes to a decrease in summer maximum temperatures.

The city has a morphology defined by the urban tissue: built-up areas, streets and alleys, green and blue areas, vacant lots. The flux of natural light and heat is conditioned by the shape, height and volume of buildings, the width of public thoroughfares, the physical and chemical properties of materials: roughness, heat conductivity and colour of stones, plastics, metal, concrete, etc. These characteristics also influence air turbulence and are thus responsible for particular microclimates. Built-up areas and roads are impervious to rain and modify the water course accordingly.

The urban edaphotope (underground, abiotic substratum) is extraordinarily diversified. Under the various pavements and tar covers lie the natural soil and sub-soil (sand, silt, clay), more or less transformed, the texture of which is important for the stability of buildings and the water course. In them are found various substrates belonging to buildings: wood, limestone or sandstone, brick, concrete, slates, asbestos sheets, metals, etc. In the paths or avenues which are not tar-covered, there is a peculiar type of soil, rich in iron scraps, soot, broken glass, tobacco butts, etc.

The soils on which vegetation grows are diverse. Large green areas such as parks or gardens generally have 'normal' soils; but under single lines of trees or in smaller green areas surrounding recent buildings, the soil is often modified physically by treading, parking of vehicles, etc., or chemically, by alkalinization. Moreover, it is full of pipes of all kind: water, electricity, telephone, gas, gutters, the leaks from which can have considerable consequences.

The water supply of the urban ecosystem is complex. Rain water soaks the ground of the green areas and flows on roofs and street surfaces, often to be dispatched to the gutter together with liquid waste. Pipes bring in drinking water from the outside. The blue areas – rivers, lakes and ponds – take part in matter and energy fluxes.

The water cycle in cities is not well known: rain is increased by condensation of vapour on the 'nuclei' of the dust dome, but evapotranspiration and percolation are reduced as the many impervious surfaces favour water run-off.

Even in the most urbanised districts, natural elements are still present: sun, air, water, plants or weeds – often not indigenous – and animals, often domestic: dogs, cats, horses, etc. An ever more intense automobile traffic brings about a new management of the urban tissue and of thoroughfares; the mood of the 'driving man' influences the whole anthropocenosis.

Another important flux is that of building materials. Every year a huge amount of them enters the city, and even more if it is a booming town or a city under reconstruction. A high flux of energy is associated with these materials, to transport and use them.

The particular feature of cities is anthropocenosis: many social or ecosociological groups mingling, cooperating or confronting one another. The study of conflicts – endogenous within social groups, exogenous between separate groups – and of their ecological causes is an important and often overlooked chapter of urban ecology (Rappoport, 1974).

City dwellers are responsible for creating their own semiotic or cultural environment. Some of the outdoor manifestations of this, such as architecture, monuments, public art, tree-lined avenues, advertising hoardings, light signs, etc., create the visual framework for their lives (Rougerie, 1975).

### *Sub-systems*

The urban ecosystem can be divided into sub-systems or districts, classified according to their social, administrative or economic roles. Urban sub-systems can be classified after Dansereau (see above), but the following area classification by Doxiadis is perhaps more practical:

- naturareas, in which what is left of wildlife is virgin, visited, embraced, invaded, or conquered;
- cultivareas: mostly horticultural zones, natural, then industrialized; note the importance of urban vegetable gardens;
- anthropareas, where people really live: the population density of built-up neighbourhoods ranges from low (about 70 h/Ha), to medium (around 110 h/Ha), to high (300 h/Ha and up);
- industriareas: heavy industry, waste disposal zones.

Along these lines, Duvigneaud et al. (1977, 1986a) have devised the mapping of the Brussels and Charleroi sub-systems in Belgium, according to the percentage of each area covered with vegetation.

## Anthropocenosis and its ecological problems

The relationship between man, health and environment is clearest in the cities. R. Abbou (1972) has studied the types of pollution and nuisances present in an urban environment and their consequences on the health of the inhabitants. According to his description, people can be affected either by their environment or by the action of other people.

In the first case, the action can be direct: physico-chemical agents, such as ionising radiation, exhaust fumes, asbestos dust, carcinogenic substances, or climatic circumstances, such as temperature, moisture and wind. It can also be indirect: visual and olfactive pollution, noise, effect of the lack of greenery. Indoor pollution must also be taken into account.

In the second case, pollution can have a biological aspect: it can be due, for example, to particle emission, contagion by germs, parasites, lice, effects of food additives or of excesses of medicines. There is also a psychosocial aspect: the stress and strain in everyday life, e.g. the car, loneliness, psychosomatic illnesses, the need to gamble, and the use and abuse of alcohol, tobacco, and hard and soft drugs.

The city is also the optimal ground for cultural intoxication, and the purposeful exploitation of crowd psychology, through, for instance, collective hysteria (rock music), too much advertising, and media intoxication.

Stress, and the presence in the environment of toxic substances or radiation to which man is not adapted – food pollution is an obvious example – induce a range of modern illnesses, from everyday afflictions such as tiredness, road or work accidents, and depression, to so-called 'civilisation diseases' – cancers, AIDS, drug dependency, reactional neuroses and psychoses. A new man is appearing, Homo circulans, who knows how to keep moving and insert himself, both in the traffic and in social life, and he has become a model for tricksters and racketeers.

## The ecological crisis: a polluted and damaged noosphere – the need for a living culture

Is man a destroyer? There are Jeremiahs, who see evil everywhere, and Panglosses, for whom 'everything is for the best in the best possible world'.

The world is suffering today from a strong imbalance, due partly to an explosive progression of science, engineering and technology, with all the risks that abuses of these can bring, such as pollution, dangers of genetic engineering or of the nuclear industry, weapons in the hands of gangsters or terrorists, etc.

However, we are witnessing too a deculturation (advertising, rock, football, gambling, rackets of all kinds, intellectual piracy) leading to generalised incompetence, encouraged by the media. There is a kind of super-informatisation excluding thought, imagination and creativity. The level of popular education is becoming lower than that of robots.

In Figure 2.2, **A** represents this anti-ecological world where renewable resources are being renewed less and less, and where non-renewable resources are more and more exhausted. Hate, conflict and economic collapse lead to a war of extermination, a nuclear winter which could mean the end of humankind.

In **B**, the alternative is a world based on a constructive ecology and on the rational use of natural resources. With this ecology in mind, the branches of culture – literary and artistic, scientific and technical – could merge into a single living culture (Lang, 1984) spread by all forms of teaching and media.

This convergence, the foundation of a renewed technology and economy, is summarised here in a heart-shaped figure emerging into a peaceful and progressive society.

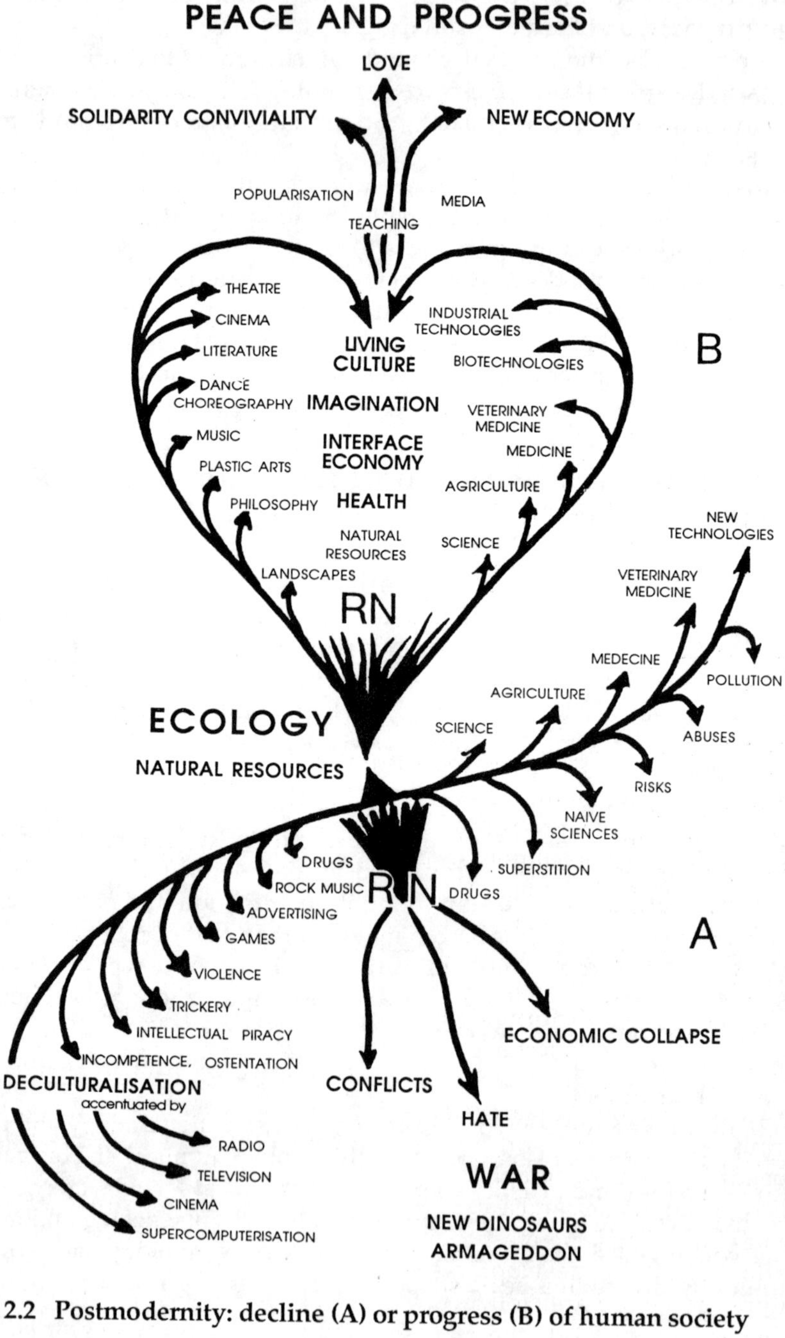


**Fig. 2.2 Postmodernity: decline (A) or progress (B) of human society**

## Post-modernity: an upgrading of the noosphere – the sophiosphere

The decline of the biosphere and the noosphere can be countered by basing ecodevelopment on constructive ecology, including human ecology.

A better balanced agrosphere would renovate the agro-sectors – food, pharmaceuticals, industry. An example would be the use of alternative cultures of new species or varieties of plants (Duvigneaud, 1986b), or integrated cultures of the SYTA type (Sustained Yield Tropical Agroecosystems) as proposed by Janzen (1973). A considerable biomass could be produced in Europe by giant weeds (often imported, and now subspontaneous), such as, in Belgium, *Polygonum cuspidatum* from Japan, *Heracleum mantegazzianum* from the Caucasus, or *Impatiens glandulifera* from the Himalayas. This biomass could provide energy or new materials for the chemical industry.

Constructive ecology can also be applied to forestry: the creation of forest ecosystems with better qualitative and quantitative yields, which would increase the possibilities of use for wood, leaves and fruits. A well-managed forest should also be used as a leisure area and as the instrument of sylvotherapy, a new and important branch of modern ecological medicine (Plaisance, 1985).

Agroforestry, a mingling of agriculture and sylviculture, exemplified in Europe by the 'bocage' – a network of hedges, lines of trees and drives giving rhythm to the rural landscape – has many ecological advantages. It is nowadays strongly advocated for tropical regions (in the SYTA frame), and should remain in the future a component of agricultural landscapes.

Another important application for ecology is the fight against desertification: reforestation, or desert agriculture (with a minimal use of fresh water, or with the use of sea water, or by seeding the soil surface with water-retaining polymers) require a sound knowledge of the fluxes, balances, and cycles of energy, water and minerals.

The use of genetic engineering and of biotechnology should not be neglected in the transformation of raw biomasses; this implies a thorough knowledge of microbiocenoses and of mycocenoses.

Constructive ecology could also be applied to urban and industrial ecosystems, the built-up areas being penetrated by natural elements (cf. Le Corbusier): sun, fresh air, blue and green areas, and peri-urban forests, depending on the topography.

Ecodevelopment, landscape ecology and teledetection are the favoured themes of a constructive ecology, but an aspect which should not be overlooked is ethnodevelopment, i.e. taking full account of living traditions, culture, homelore and folklore. Marrying development and culture, or trying to restore both the ecology and the culture of degraded areas, becomes an ever more important problem in land use planning (Eilart, 1988; Janzen, 1988).

For a holistic approach to the human environment, Barret (1981) suggested as a basic unit the noosystem, which has a wider meaning than the ecosystem since it includes the social, economic and cultural influences on the ecosystem. This noosystem should be managed by using problem-solving algorithms, in a way which allows the 'applied ecologist' to take scientific decisions about resource management. systematically.

But modern man, instead of applying his mind and reason to the numerous possible types of eco- and ethnodevelopment, behaves like an industrialized, deculturized predator. He destroys his environment; he increases the human population beyond the carrying capacity, and well beyond the cultural capacity; he over-exploits, and often wastes natural resources, renewable or not; soils are degraded and exhausted. Man has a thousand ways of polluting and destroying his environment and his health, of inventing and accumulating deadly chemical, bacteriological or nuclear weapons. Fear sets in. Bound in a society that demands maximum profits, man loses and forgets his personality and turns into an anonymous, fanaticized or zombified being (Finkielkraut, 1987). Driven by conflicts often rooted in the man-made environment (Rappoport, 1974), mankind is running headlong towards its own undoing and the extinction of the species. We are the new dinosaurs.

Many voices have already uttered such pessimistic conclusions: from the 'Armageddon' of the Bible and the American ecologists, to the 'Mégamort' of E. Morin (1984), the threat of a new Hitler (Toynbee, 1971), the decline into barbarianism (Henry, 1987). To stop this decline and develop a new autonomy within conviviality, man has to change.[2] Hope would lie in a new ecological morality,[3] which is conceivable only as a synthesis of the various fields of interest for the human mind (in the sense of Diderot and D'Alembert).

This new morality would embody the meeting of scientific and humanistic cultures, often called for and never realised.[4] A living culture, based on a natural environment and its resources, rooted in the past and its psychological permanence, linking regional and universal scales, could emerge in arts and techniques which would allow man's needs to be satisfied and ensure him a good quality of life, in a noosphere where the economy, the exploitation of resources, the social structure and the distribution of wealth would be kept in balance.

---

[2] Huyghe, 1987, Rappoport, 1974; Illich 1973; Grandstedt, 1980; Peccei, 1976.

[3] Alsopp, 1972; Duvigneaud, 1972; Dubos, 1974; Saint-Marc, 1978.

[4] Prigogine and Stengers, 1979; Prigogine, 1988.

Is this Utopia or a possible reality for tomorrow? Will the sophiosphere (sphere of wisdom) replace a noosphere where man's intelligence has all too often been in the service of evil?

## References


Abbou, R., *Médecine écologique*, Paris, 1972.

Alsopp, B., *Ecological morality*, F. Muller, London, 1972.

Barret, G.W., 'Stress ecology, an integrative approach' in Barret, G.W. and Rosenberg, R., *Stress effects in natural ecosystems*, John Wiley, New York, 1981, pp. 3–12.

Dansereau, P., 'Essai de classification et de cartographie écologique des espaces', *Etudes écologiques*, vol. 10, Université du Québec, Montréal, 1985.

Doxiadis, C.A., *Ecology and ekistics*, Elek, London, 1977.

Dubos, R., *Choisir d'être humain*, Denoël, Paris, 1974.

Duvigneaud, P., *Morale et écologie*, La Pensée et les Hommes, Bruxelles, 1972.

Duvigneaud, P., Denayer, S., Brichard, C. and C., Bouchat, A., Moniquet, J.C. and Chasseur, C., *Les composantes de l'écosystème Charleroi et les prospectives de développement socio-économique régional*, Bur. Econ. Hainaut, Mons, 1986a.

Duvigneaud, P., Denayer, S., De Smet, S. and Tanghe, M., *Carte écologique de l'occupation du sol et des degrés de verdurisation de l'agglomération bruxelloise*, Agglom. de Bruxelles, Service de l'Environnement, 1977.

Duvigneaud, P., Moniquet, J.C. and Brichard, Ch., *Culture du tournesol, culture artistique et avenir de la Wallonie*, Bur. Econ. Hainaut, Mons, 1986b.

Eilart, J., *Man, ecosystems and culture*, Perioditia, Tallinn (Estonia), 1976.

Ellenberg, H., 'Bäuerliche Bauweisen in geoökologischer und genetischer Sicht', *Geogr. Zeitschrift*, H.7, F. Steiner, Stuttgart, 1984, p. 69.

Finkielkraut, A., *La défaite de la pensée*, Gallimard, Paris, 1987.

Grandstedt, I., *L'impasse industrielle*, Seuil, Paris, 1980.

Haekel, E., 'Über Entwicklungsgang und Aufgabe der Zoologie', *Jenaische Zeitschrift.*, vol. 5, pp. 353–70.

Hardin, G., 'Cultural carrying capacity: a biological approach to human problems', *Bioscience*, vol. 36, no. 9, 1986, pp. 599–606.

Henry, M., *La barbarie*, Grasset, Paris, 1987.

Huyghe, F.B., *La soft idéologie*, Laffont, Paris, 1987.

Illich, I., *La convivialité*, Seuil, Paris, 1973.

Janzen, D.H., 'Tropical Agroecosystems', *Science*, vol. 142, pp. 1212–19, 1973.

Janzen, D.H., 'Tropical ecological and biocultural restoration', *Science*, vol. 239, 1988, pp. 243–4.

Jouret, B., *Définition spatiale du phénomène urbain bruxellois*, Ed. Univ. Bruxelles, 1977.

Lang, J., cited by Dickson, D., 'France puts Diderot in the limelight', *Science*, 1984, pp. 1132–3.

Lapo, A.V., *Traces of bygone biospheres*, Mir, Moscow, 1987.

Morin, E., *Pour sortir du Vingtième siècle*, Seuil, Paris, 1984.

Plaisance, G., *Forêt et santé: guide pratique et sylvothérapie*, Dangles, St. Jean de Braye, 1985.

Peccei, A., *La qualité humaine*, Stock, Paris, 1976.

Prigogine, I., 'Une nouvelle alliance de la science et de la culture', *Courrier de l'UNESCO*, May 1988, pp. 9–13.

Prigogine, I. and Stengers, I., *La nouvelle alliance*, Gallimard, Paris, 1979.

Rappoport, A., *Conflict in man-made environments*, Pelican, 1974.

Reiter, H., *Konsolidation des Physiognomik als Versuch einer Ökologie der Gewächse*, Graz, 1885.

Rougerie, G., *Les cadres de vie*, P.U.F., Paris, 1975.

Saint-Marc, P., *Progrès ou déclin de l'homme*, Stock, Paris, 1978.

Sorre, M., *Les fondements de la géographie humaine, I. Les fondements biologiques, Essai d'une écologie de l'homme*, A. Collin, Paris, 1947.

Teilhard de Chardin, P., *La place de l'homme dans la nature*, A. Michel, Paris, 1956.

Toynbee, A., *Surviving the Future*, Oxford University Press, 1971.

Vernadsky, W., *La Géochimie*, Alcan, Paris, 1924.

Vernadsky, W., *La biosphère*, Alcan, Paris, 1929.

Vernadsky, W., 'The biosphere and the noosphere', *American Scientist*, vol. 33, no. 1, pp. 8–9, 1945.

Chapter 3

# A survey of the dangers of the chemical era: impacts on human and environmental health

by René Truhaut

One of the essential characteristics of our age has certainly been the prodigious development of the chemical industry and the consequent continuous spread of the use of chemicals in widely differing domains.

The spectacular progress in chemical science has played an essential role in our contemporary world and brought enormous benefits both economically and socially. But, as always, there is another side to the coin, and it is important not to forget the risk of harm that can result from human exposure, in the course of modern life, to a large and constantly growing number of chemicals, some of which are hazardous to health. This poses problems for toxicologists, hygienists, doctors, safety engineers and technologists as to what measures to take to protect the population against these hazards.

This chapter draws attention to the dangers that can result from the chemical era and to the general principles of prevention that should be applied to prevent, or at least to reduce, the dangers as much as possible.

## Different kinds of toxicity

The first kind of toxicity to consider is acute or sub-acute toxicity , i.e., the toxicity which results immediately or a short time after the absorption all at once or in closely spaced intervals of a sufficiently large dose of the chemical being considered. This happens following the ingestion of many substances, penetration of the skin or inhalation in the case of gas or fumes such as carbon monoxide, chloride or cyanide. The appearance of this form of toxicity is dramatic since it can lead rapidly to death.

Toxic effects result not only from the absorption in a short space of time of relatively large doses, but also very often from a much more insidious form of poisoning that generally occurs without warning. This is long-term toxicity, which results from the accumulation of doses or the summation of effects.

The absorption of small doses of so-called cumulative toxins that would be without noticeable consequence if they were eliminated normally, will, after a time, lead to a toxic threshold concentration being reached in the target organ or tissue, causing disorders in which the symptoms are highly variable.

Substances having carcinogenic effects seem to be even more dangerous. From results obtained using an azo dye which produces tumours in rats, Druckrey and Kupfmuller (1949) developed the paradoxical idea that the effects of each isolated dose were added during the entire life of the experimental animal no matter what elimination and metabolic degradation took place. Thus there would be not only an accumulation of the doses but a total summation of absolutely irreversible effects. This concept has evolved somewhat as there are several categories of carcinogens which differ in the way they act. For certain of these it has been possible to fix thresholds, but it is not possible here to go into more detail about these.

In the past few years, different examples have been provided of substances that provoke serious effects in animals or humans after a more or less prolonged latent phase and after its elimination from the organism. The herbicide Paraquat, a derivative of bipyridinium, is an example. Several weeks after ingestion of a dose that only causes minor gastro-intestinal problems, a proliferation of fibroblasts on the pulmonary epithelium can cause death through inhibition of oxygen diffusion. These are, as John Barnes called them, 'poisons that hit and run'.

Much interest is attached to the study of effects on reproductive functions and especially embryotoxic effects. Among these, teratogenetic effects (birth defects) are a special case which will be referred to again later. Mutagenic effects – the production of mutations and other special effects (e.g. immunosuppression, effects on behaviour, sensitisation and many other, sometimes subtle, effects) – must also be mentioned.

These different categories of effects illustrate the multiplicity of the methodological approaches needed to evaluate the toxic potential of environmental pollutants.

## Risks for human health from exposure to chemicals

*Drugs.* It is well known that a chemical which has beneficial properties at certain doses justifying a therapeutic use, can, at higher doses or over a longer period of time, cause symptoms of toxicity even at the same target site as the therapeutic effects are felt. But the problem of secondary effects of medicines on other targets is by far the most studied of therapeutic risks. The case of medicines is special, since the prescribing doctor has to weigh up the benefits against the risks.

*Chemicals in the workplace.* Of course it is proper to worry about acute or even sometimes mass poisonings that can result from accidental exposure to high doses of toxic substances, especially volatile substances. But much more often, exposure to small doses of substances with a cumulative toxic effect, day after day in industrial workplaces, causes long-term poisoning of the workers. As early as 1703 the great Italian doctor, Bernardino Ramazzini, wrote: 'Artisans frequently find serious illness in the very place where they hoped to find the means to feed their families, and they die cursing the occupation that they chose.'

*Chemicals in food.* The ever-increasing use of chemicals in food and agriculture means that many substances are incorporated:

- by treatment preceding the slaughter of animals or the harvest of comestible plants;
- by contamination during processing, storage or distribution;
- by intentional introduction of chemicals for various reasons: preservation; improvement of smell, taste, appearance, presentation, etc.

The study of the risks of damage that can result from the presence of these substances in food is one of the great current problems of toxicology. It cannot be stressed too strongly, in view of the fact that people are fatally subjected to the influence of their food from birth to death.

*Air pollution.* Air is the most essential element to sustain life. A human individual absorbs each day from birth to death about twelve cubic metres or a bit more than fifteen kilos. All adulteration of its purity is therefore of primary importance. Sufficiently small particles can penetrate to the pulmonary alveoli where they can produce harmful effects, but also can pass into the circulatory system.

*Chemicals in the home.* Apart from specifically domestic products, many of which carry risks to health if rigorous precautions are not observed (e.g. cleaning and housekeeping products and insecticides), cosmetics and toiletries are important to consider if they could be partially ingested. For example, certain colouring agents used for lipstick, such as rhodamine B, are considered to be potentially carcinogenic.

## Risks to the environment

But the human race is not alone in the universe. We form a part of ecosystems, or biotopes, inhabited by communities of micro-organisms, plants and animals in equilibrium with each other and their environment. Although they each have autonomy, ecosystems – whether terrestrial or aquatic – have reciprocal relationships and interact harmoniously so as to form a coherent whole on the surface of the earth: the biosphere.

In this context of biological equilibrium, the study of the harmful effects of chemicals (usually of human origin) on the various components of the biosphere has enormous importance. To define this new branch of science was the fundamental objective of the new branch of toxicology which we proposed in June, 1969, during a meeting of an ad hoc committee of the International Council of Scientific Unions (ICSU) in Stockholm. We gave it the name of Ecotoxicology.

We quickly realized that a more elaborate definition of ecotoxicology was needed to differentiate this specialised branch from its mother discipline of classical toxicology. Although the latter studies toxic effects in individual organisms, ecotoxicology studies their impact on populations of living organisms which make up the ecosystem, from human beings to micro-organisms.

Ecotoxicological studies cover three main sequences of events which are, especially in the case of (1) and (2) most often interlinked:

(1) Emission and entry of pollutants into the physical environment with a study of their distribution and their fate;
(2) Entry and fate of pollutants in the biological environment with the very important problem of the contamination of biological chains and, foremost, food chains;
(3) Qualitative and quantitative study of toxic effects of chemical pollutants with an examination of the impact upon humans.

### *Entry of pollutants into the environment*

Each year some 500 new chemical compounds are put on the market and added to the approximately 27,000 currently in use (Stanford Research Institute). The main sources of emissions are: domestic and industrial heating and generators; industrial effluents; motor vehicles, ships and planes using petroleum or inorganic oil fuels; industrial products for a whole series of purposes (e.g. asbestos, PCBs, solvents, various wood preservatives, nuclear fuels); agricultural chemicals; and household and domestic products (solvents, detergents, paint, varnish, insecticides, medicines, cosmetics, plastic packaging, detergents – and their many additives).

Air emissions are important, not only for gas and fumes, but also for particles – especially those small enough to be dispersed in the form of aerosols which can be transported over long distances. These particles, besides their own potentially toxic properties, can play a very important role either as carriers of gas and fumes, or as supporting elements for catalytic alterations which possibly generate harmful compounds. Atmospheric pollutants are also liable to provide fall-out which then pollutes the upper layer of the soil as well as the plants growing there. Such is the case for numerous pesticides used in agriculture, metal derivatives of fluoride, and metal derivatives of lead formed during the combustion of organic compounds of lead in high-octane fuels.

## *Distribution of chemicals in the environment*

After entering the physical environment, pollutants are subjected to a whole range of factors liable to influence their distribution. Various meteorological conditions, such as wind, rain, fog or temperature inversions, play a part. Pollutants can be transformed, giving rise to new compounds. A striking example is the formation of irritant and phytotoxic peracyl nitrates (an element of smog) from components of car exhaust and aeroplane reactors by photochemical reactions due to solar radiation.

There are large lacunae in our knowledge concerning the fate of numerous chemical pollutants of the environment. We do not know what happens to carbon monoxide in car exhaust, to the tonnes of trichloroethylene released when this solvent is used in dry cleaning textiles, or to the contraceptives (or their metabolites) excreted by millions of women taking these drugs?

## *Fate of pollutants in the environment*

This could be called the 'chemico-bio-kinetics' of pollutants in ecosystems if we consider the latter as 'supraspecific organisms'. Research includes studies on the absorption, distribution and fate of pollutants in biological chains with the possibilities of accumulation in one link or another or metabolic alteration and reactions with chemical constituents of the living organisms which make up the biological chains. The means of absorption depends both on the nature of the living organisms and on the nature of the substrate in which they live.

Beside the concentrations in organisms, much interest is attached to the study of selective accumulations within a given species in some organs or tissues. It is important to establish the critical concentrations and the rhythm of detoxification, and the biological half-life of persistent pollutants.

## *Metabolic alteration of chemicals*

Pollutants, once they have entered living organisms, find themselves in contact with enzyme systems that can make them undergo metabolic alterations. These alterations, which use a series of biochemical processes, can be classified as biodegradation or metabolic transformation.. Biodegradation means that the alterations result in products less toxic than the molecules from which they are derived, causing a detoxification of the latter.

Metabolic transformation can also cause alterations that give rise to compounds which are more toxic than the molecules from which they are derived. A classical example of such toxifying transformations is the alteration of nitrates, from the nitrogen cycle or from fertilizer, under the influence of denitrifying bacteria to form nitrites.

Certain molecules undergo practically no metabolic change; they are so little soluble in water and so very soluble in lipids that they have a tendency to accumulate in living organisms. For example, the levels of certain insecticides or polychlorinated biphenyls (PCBs) in certain aquatic organisms can reach values 10,000 times higher than those found in the water in which the organisms live.

## *Damage to the biosphere*

Biological effects on the constituents of ecosystems from chemical pollution can indirectly have an impact on people. Some examples are:

- Reduction in food resources caused by episodes of pollution:
  - mass killings of fish by toxic waste water discharged into waters;
  - unfavourable biological conditions for aquatic food species, created by the depletion of oxygen resulting from excessive eutrophication with respect to plant species (notably algae) following the influx in excessive quantities of inorganic salts such as phosphates;
  - damage to crops from air pollution, such as oxidising photochemical smog;
- Indirect effects on agricultural productivity following toxic effects on beneficial organisms such as bees or earthworms;
- Toxification of elements of food chains:
  - contamination of fish by derivatives of methylmercury;
  - storage in mammalian milk of different residues of lipo-soluble, organo-chlorinated pesticides, metabolites of aflatoxins or radioactive fission products;

- Production of pathogenic bacteria having resistance to antibiotics;
- Loss of productivity of raw materials, such as textile plants or forest plantations;
- Disruption of biological equilibria in nature with consequent loss of the recreational possibilities.

## *Factors which influence toxicity or damage*

Numerous factors exert an influence on the qualitative and quantitative nature of toxicity. Two of the most important are the species involved and the developmental stage.

***Species.*** It is well known that for the majority of chemical agents there are big variations in receptivity to their toxic effects according to the species considered. This is one of the big difficulties in evaluating the toxic potentials in human toxicology because extrapolation to humans of results obtained in experimentation on laboratory animals carries a lot of uncertainties. It is for this reason that so much importance is given to completing the results from experimental toxicology with observations on groups of humans exposed,. Particularly during the course of an epidemiological investigation, one needs objective clinical as well as biological criteria.

A good illustration of this fact is found among the organo-phosphorous insecticides. Malathion, for example, is 150 to 200 times less toxic for mammals than parathion, while being practically as toxic to most insects. There is still much to be learned in this area.

***Developmental stage.*** This is a very important factor because of the frequency of hypersensitivity of embryonic forms and during the first stages of life. In human toxicology, it is now a classical concept that the foetus is particularly sensitive to toxic attack, especially at the stage of organogenesis. The study of these effects, called *teratogenetic,* has therefore been included in the protocol for toxicological experiments for all drugs. It must be stressed that teratogenetic effects are only one example of embryotoxic effects which sometimes can appear over a long period and sometimes over a *very* long period.

The importance of prenatal toxicology must be taken into careful consideration with respect to professional, industrial or agricultural exposure. Infants and young children are also very sensitive to the toxic potential of chemicals. This hypersensitivity stems from different factors including metabolic immaturity and deficiencies in detoxifying enzymes. In ecotoxicology, the possibility of toxic attack on the first stages of life – particularly larval forms, such as fish fry and bird embryos – are, it would seem, very important for the propagation of the species.

## General principles of prevention

One can only really guard against the dangers that one knows about. This is why the main principal of prevention against the dangers of the chemical era is the discovery and disclosure of toxic risks. As in human toxicology, the ultimate objective of ecotoxicological research must be the establishment of protective measures against harmful effects of environmental pollutants on the different constituents of ecosystems and biological equilibria.

Thus, it is necessary to implement an adequate methodology for toxicological evaluation. We would also like to emphasize the interest and importance that has been connected for the past few years to the efforts to develop test methods on *in vitro* systems in order to limit as much as possible the use of laboratory animals. A certain number of approaches, such as studies on cell cultures and in particular hepatocytes, have proved extremely fertile. Attention must be given to the study of possible long-term risks because people are exposed throughout their entire lives to chemical agents in the environment and in food.

### *The types of tests*

By reason of the uncertainty that always accompanies the extrapolation to humans of results obtained using experimental animals and in the tests on *in vitro* systems, the ideal method would be to experiment directly on humans. For both practical and moral reasons, this cannot be done except in very special cases.

In this respect, it cannot be overemphasized that our qualitative and particularly our quantitative information is still very limited as far as ecotoxic effects are concerned. Even if we restrict ourselves to the study of aquatic ecosystems, which are the object of study at the national and international level (Ecotoxicology Section of the Scientific Committee of the EC on the Toxicity and Ecotoxicity of Chemicals), the available data concern, in fact, only a certain number of species (Daphnia, certain fishes), and they are restricted for the most part to results of acute or sub-acute toxicity because only fairly rarely are data on chronic toxicity available. For the determination of criteria for the quality of aquatic environments as well as toxicity, one must take into consideration two other parameters: persistence linked to the absence of biodegradability and bioaccumulation at certain levels in biological chains.

The multiplicity of the problems to study requires coordination of research on a global scale within the context of multidisciplinary cooperation. This would require the participation of specialists from a whole series of disciplines, particularly the various branches of ecology and until now have often pursued their studies without seeking to exchange information on their methods and results.

It is also indispensable, we wish to repeat, that specialists in the science of analysis should be associated with this work. How, in fact, to establish the relationships between dose and its response without having available adequately sensitive and specific methods to measure the exposure doses? How to study the fate of a pollutant in the physical environment, its movement, and that of its possible degradation products through ecosystems without having available precise techniques for identification and dosage in complex biological environments made up of biological chains where pollutants and the products of their metabolic transformation are in general considerably diluted?

## *Prevention*

A number of general principles that can lead to the utilisation of technical measures for the prevention of risks from chemicals have been revealed through our research over the past years.

*Avoidance of highly dangerous substances.* The ideal principle would be to avoid products that are too dangerous. It is easily applied in the case of drugs such as thalidomide, additives such as bromacetates, pesticides such as organo-chlorine derivatives, or industrial products with a highly carcinogenic activity such as beta-propiolactone or nitrosamines.

But this principle cannot be applied in such an absolute way to the air pollutants of a city. It is hard to see how to completely eliminate benzo(a)pyrene in regions with a lot of traffic. It is appropriate therefore to reduce as much as possible the quantity of pollutants released by the progressive introduction of adequate technical means. In the case of very toxic industrial products, effects must be made to replace them with products that are functionally equivalent and that are, if not completely harmless, at least of a very feeble toxicity. A dramatic example in this direction is that of the progressive replacement of benzene as an industrial solvent by products like toluene, cyclohexane and the chlorine derivatives of ethylene.

*The exclusion of impurities.* It is important to remember that very often the toxicity of a substance can be due to impurities it contains. It is well known, for example, that trichloroethylene used to be much more toxic than it is now. The corollary for regulation is obviously to establish standards of purity. Such a measure should be applied particularly rigorously to food additives.

*Labelling dangerous chemicals.* It is important that people are warned about known toxic risks from chemicals. With good reason this problem of labelling is preoccupying many national authorities and international organisations like the World Health Organization, the United Nations Environment Programme, the International Labour Organisation and the Council of Europe.

*Finding antidotes and making them known.* In the face of growing numbers of accidental poisonings, it is necessary to assemble information on emergency therapeutic measures, particularly the antidotes to use.

*Setting concentration limits for dangerous substances in the workplace.* The major means of controlling hazards is, after having fixed a threshold of toxicity, to establish tolerable concentration limits for which and below which there is practically no danger either from short exposure (ceiling values) or from long-term exposure, or, when it is a cumulative poison, of repeated exposure day after day even in conditions of industrial or agricultural work (time-weighted averages). What we consider to be the golden rule of toxicology – set out five centuries ago by Paracelsus – is applicable both to the case of substances being intentionally or unintentionally absorbed, and to toxicity in the workplace: 'Dose makes the poison.'

*Compiling positive lists, particularly for food additives.* A 'positive' list should be established containing the names of chemicals and their acceptable concentrations. The fundamental toxicological fact for each product conforming to the doctrine that we presented in 1957 to the Sub-Committee for the Health and Safety of Food of the Council of Europe. This has been unanimously adopted on an international scale; it is known as the acceptable daily intake (ADI) for prolonged absorption. From this one can, taking into account the maximum permissible level of consumption of the food under consideration, calculate the maximum permissible concentration and even fix tolerance levels which, in conditions of good food technology or good agricultural practice, can be considerably lower.

*Setting and controlling standards for chemical assessment.* It is practically useless to adopt standards if adequate analytical methods of measurement and control are not available. This is an enormous field of activity where the International Union of Pure and Applied Chemistry (IUPAC) has a considerable role to play in cooperating with other international organisations and the European Community.

*Health education, especially for chemists.* An important action would be the promotion of adequate health education – not only for people exposed to chemicals but also for the managers of the chemical industry, who are often unaware of the long-term dangers of their products. For this reason, it seems highly desirable to include in the teaching of chemistry a part devoted to the presentation of the fundamental concepts of toxicology.

## Conclusions

In this survey I have only been able to give some very general and therefore very incomplete insights into the vast subject which is the science of toxicology and ecotoxicology. Nevertheless, I hope to have shown the dangers to health and to biological equilibria in the environment that chemicals can cause if careful attention is not given to the prior assessment of their risks by adequate toxicological studies which provide a basis for preventive measures.

It is highly desirable to develop global centres of toxicological and ecotoxicological research to apply the multi-disciplinary methods that are needed. It cannot be over emphasised how underdeveloped the science of toxicology is, even in the most advanced countries such as the United States. This is even more true in the case of ecotoxicology, despite its very fruitful research so far.

Moreover, the time is gone when the objectives of toxicology were limited to only certain fields. It is a science whose fundamental objective is to protect the health of the population as well as the quality of their environment and thus to enable them to enjoy the benefits of progress of modern chemistry in complete safety. This is a particularly exalting objective for all who are engaged in this field of research.

Chapter 4

# Evaluating persistent pollutants in the environment

by Friedhelm Korte and Mohammed Mansour

The expression 'environmental chemicals' has arisen because the vast majority of synthetic, man-made substances are persistent: they spread out all over the world and become omnipresent. To reduce the potential hazards of chemicals we need to know their effects on human beings as well as the effects on animals, plants, terrestrial and aquatic ecosystems and materials. For this we need to have accurate information about the chemicals' behaviour and fate in the different environmental compartments: air, soil and water.

The lifetimes of organic chemicals in the environment are determined by chemical processes. Reactions in the compartments – for example, oxidations initiated by sunlight – are known to change the concentrations of organic compounds, leading to their ultimate degradation. Thus it is necessary to know which chemical processes dominate in each compartment.

Chemicals can enter the environment in any of the three compartments. Subsequent distribution depends on the chemical's physico-chemical properties. By measuring vapour pressure, water solubility, volatility, adsorption, desorption[1], and dispersion, one can predict in which

[1] Adsorption is holding molecules of a gas, liquid or soluble substances to the surface; desorption is release of a substance from the surface.

compartment the chemical is most likely to be found. Such predictions are useful in estimating which transformation may be most important for that chemical and thus which laboratory studies should be given the most consideration, the most information and data for comparative evaluation. It is critical to hazard assessment, to improve the ability to extrapolate from laboratory test results, to predict accurately and quantitatively degradation, transformation, accumulation and transport in the field.

Chemicals enter the environment and target organisms (including humans) through complex and interrelated pathways. Some chemicals – such as DDT, hexachlorobenzene, aldrin and pesticides – enter the environment through direct or indirect application. Thus the general population is constantly exposed to many chemicals. The pathways of organic chemicals from the environment to humans are summarised in Figure 4.1.

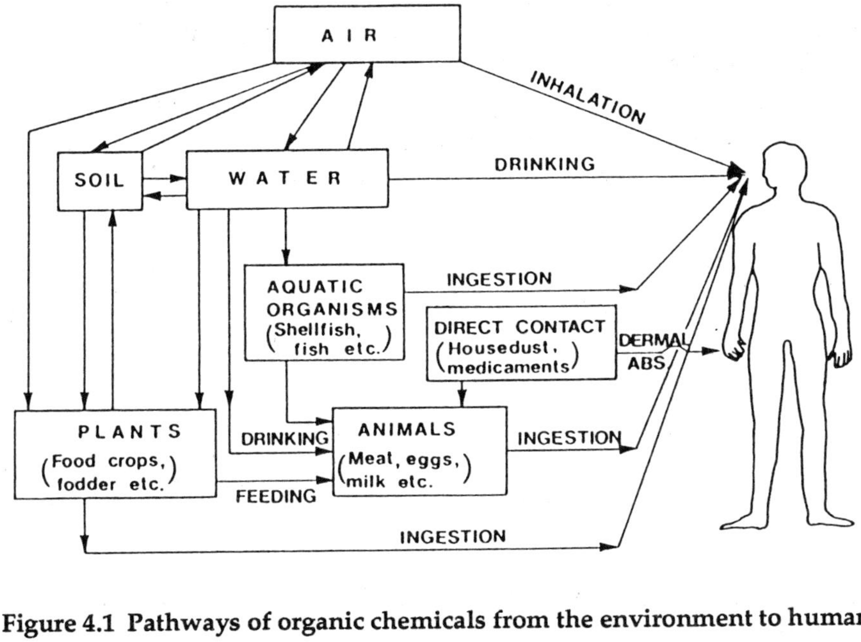


**Figure 4.1 Pathways of organic chemicals from the environment to humans**

A significant part of the assessment of chemicals today is concerned with how to establish criteria to judge environmental pollution by chemicals and how to minimise that pollution. Chemicals are useful and necessary in many cases, but hazardous in some others – and nobody can deny that both features are inseparably connected. Thus the ever growing use of chemicals in our society demands considerable action.

The aim now is to establish a sound risk/benefit correlation to evaluate a chemical's potential environmental impact. But the standards of acceptability must be dynamic rather than static, as they have to cope with changing environmental conditions and any progress made in environmental research. Recently several organisations have addressed themselves to the complex problem of overall environmental risk assessment of both existing and new chemicals, and have proposed a systematic approach based on information observed from laboratory experiments.

In principle there are two ways to approach this kind of evaluation: monitoring and predicting. With monitoring, one waits for the chemical's effects to occur and manifest themselves, and then observes and measures them. The risk here is that the damage has already begun.

To *predict* a chemical's environmental behaviour, one has to answer three basic questions:

- How and where does the chemical enter the environment?
- In which compartments of the environment does it accumulate?
- Which are the pathways of elimination?

But in order to answer these questions, we must first establish a number of parameters on which to base evaluation standards which can be applied generally. At the very least, we need the six parameters given below.

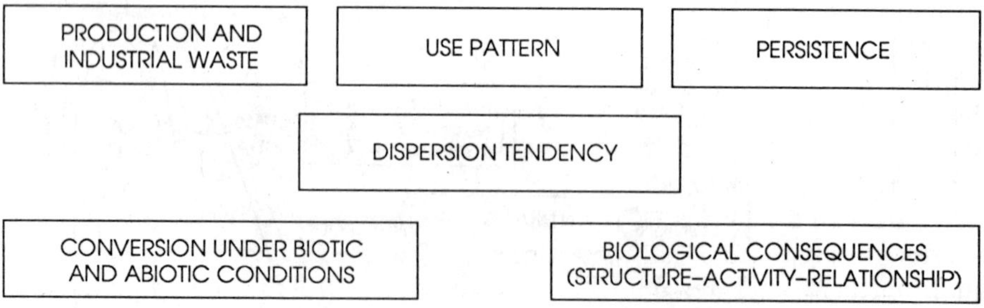


## How and where chemicals enter the environment

The quantities and sources of chemicals being released into the environment, and their regional and global concentrations, are mainly determined by production and usage patterns. In 1950, world production of synthetic organic chemicals amounted to 7 million tons; by 1970 it had reached 63 million tons; confirmed estimates for 1985 were close to 250 million tons. The European Commission's European Inventory of Existing

Commercial Chemical Substances (EINECS, 1987–88) listed 110,000 chemicals being produced and marketed in Europe by 18 September 1981.

A great variety of test methods and environmental models have been developed to try to understand the ecological significance of a chemical's ecotoxicological behaviour, its conversion under various conditions and the related elimination mechanisms. While these are highly dependent on the physical properties and structure of a chemical, they are not always dependent on its concentration. Substances which occur in almost negligible proportions today (about 1μg/kg) may reach global concentrations of about 1mg/kg in 100 years – an ecological significance that equals that of PCBs!

Although comprehensive ecotoxicological assessment is still in its very early stages, two experimental approaches have crystallised in recent years. One is based on reducing overall ecological systems to their simplest form and then, from experimentation, drawing conclusions about the behaviour of chemicals in the environment.

The second method tries to define isolated factors which govern the behaviour of chemicals within ecological systems. These factors are then investigated using experimental designs which come close to conditions encountered in practice. In our experimental investigations, we gave the second method preference as we tried to build up the concept of an ecotoxicological profile analysis.[2]

The environmental significance of chemicals is determined by the amount used, the pattern of use, the ecotoxic action, the degradability, the formation (biological and abiotic) of derivative products, the dispersion tendency, the accumulation and the behaviour of derivative products. Short-term testing cannot be expected to yield detailed information about the total behaviour of a chemical in a complex ecological system of the overall biosphere. But it should provide individual data about the chemical in selected, limited and important compartments of the environment.

We designed a series of six individual short-term test systems to give results and conclusions matching as closely as possible – at least qualititatively – the results of long-term tests with complex systems and analytical environmental investigations (see Figure 4.2).

1. Mammalian metabolism: testing in rats represents the behaviour of chemicals in warm-blooded animals;
2. Bioaccumulation: tests on fish and algae represent the behaviour of chemicals in animal, plant and microbial life of the aquatic system.

---

2 This was conceived exclusively as a way to establish priority lists for more detailed – and costly – experimental investigations; it was not intended to serve as a testing methodology for legislative measures.

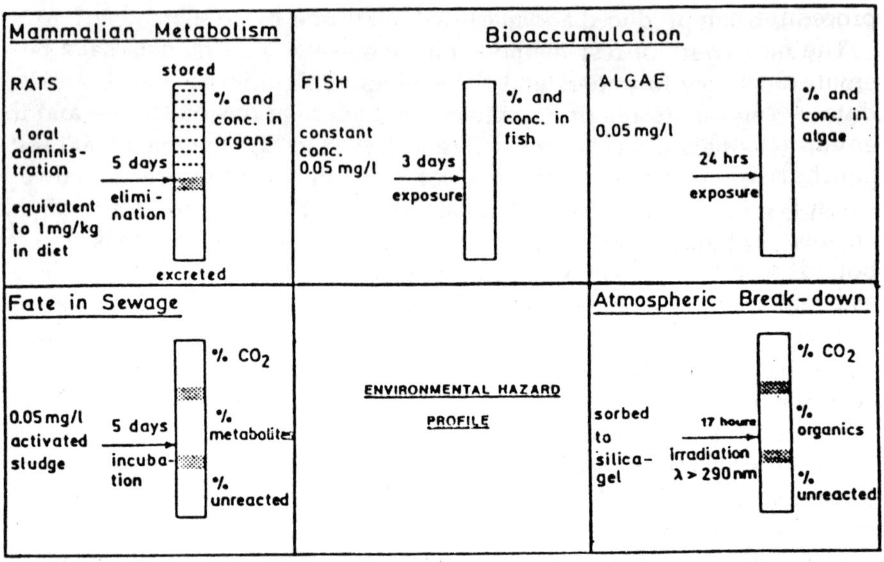


**Figure 4.2 Survey of the testing system for ecotoxicologic profile analysis** ***(All tests with*** $^{14}$***C-labelled chemicals. Evaluation to be based on a reference compound.)***

3. Fate in sewage: the activated sludge test indicates a chemical's behaviour during biological sewage treatment;[3]
4. Waste composting: the refuse composting test shows the chemical's behaviour in terms of a technique of re-using waste and also includes aspects of soil microbial degradation;
5. Waste incineration: testing by incineration gives data about the chemical's behaviour during this process and especially about its reactivity and thermal stability;
6. Atmospheric breakdown: photomineralization also represents a test of a chemical's stability and is an important criterion of abiotic (atmospheric) degradation.

Thus this system of tests investigates problems of accumulation, distribution, transformation and/or the degree of degradability of chemicals in the environment. The tests are in part related to more complex, long-term investigations, but the experimental procedure has been suitably simplified for the requirements of the profile analysis. Thus by their very

[3] Where we already know chemicals can cause massive damage.

nature the tests substantially fulfil the requirements of simplicity, rapid procedure, capacity for standardisation and low cost.

The factors embraced in the test series should reflect the most varied environmental effects possible on the chemical being studied. Individual data should indicate a relative estimate of the chemical's overall environmental behaviour when compared to the data for a reference or benchmark chemical whose environmental properties are wellknown from extensive long-term tests and analytical data. The chosen benchmark chemical should be one that is judged 'just compatible', or just within the bounds of acceptability. Then one can designate the newly tested chemical as being 'more' or 'less' environmentally compatible as the benchmark. The test series of all of the chemicals studied should be evaluated jointly in order to grade the chemicals in a priority list for more extensive and costly investigations.

We cannot emphasise strongly enough the need to develop simple laboratory tests that are reliable and highly predictive. The test system presented here provides one procedure for achieving a comparative and systematic evaluation of chemicals. But it must be recognised that any screening system, however feasible or sophisticated, will never provide reliable answers to *all* environmental questions. Thus the selection of a small number of important tests can only be one part of the ecotoxicological cost-benefit assessment of environmental chemicals.

Chapter 5

# The effects of environmental pollutants on the immune system: experimental evidence and field observations

by J.G. Vos, H. Van Loveren, P.W. Wester and A.D. Vethaak

An increase in infectious diseases in humans and in various wildlife populations has been partly attributed to exposure to environmental pollutants. Such infections can be secondary to other conditions, such as shifts in population densities, or a more favourable environment to infectious organisms. But the infections can also be the direct result of a suppression, induced by environmental chemicals, of the host's defence immune system.

Immunotoxicology is the branch of science that studies changes in defence mechanisms that are caused by chemicals and drugs. A key interest of this discipline is to evaluate such effects observed during toxicity testing in rodents in order to assess the risks for humans.

During the past decade toxicological research has indicated that the immune system, on which defence mechanisms depend, is a potential target for many chemicals foreign to the body. In experimental animals, toxicological effects of chemicals on the immune system may show up as changes in the weight and microscopic appearance of lymphoid organs (such as thymus, spleen and lymph nodes), in altered numbers of blood leukocytes, and in the impairment of immune cell functions. Such toxicity may result in an increased incidence of infectious disease or in the development of certain tumours.

The impact that suppression of the immune system can have on humans is shown by the association between use of immunosuppressive agents and an increased incidence of infectious and neoplastic diseases. For example, patients who have received a kidney transplant and who were thereafter chronically treated with immunosuppressive drugs (such as corticosteroids) show a very high frequency of secondary cancer (Penn, 1987). The consequences of immunosuppression are further illustrated both by the increased incidence of leukemias and lymphomas (tumours of lymphoid tissue) in patients with congenital immunodeficiencies, and by the opportunistic infections and Kaposi's sarcomas (a type of malignant tumour) in patients with acquired immunodeficiency syndrome, AIDS (Centers for Disease Control, 1988).

Although many chemicals are known to be immunotoxic in animal models, relatively little is known about the consequences to humans of exposure to lower levels of environmental chemicals over long time periods. One reason for this discrepancy is that there have only been a few epidemiological studies of exposed human populations. Research on polychlorinated biphenyls or PCBs is a notable exception. One such study is the investigation of so-called Yu-Cheng patients poisoned in 1979 in Taiwan by the consumption of rice oil accidentally contaminated with PCBs and polychlorinated dibenzofurans (PCDFs). These patients suffered from skin lesions, liver damage and an altered immune function (Chang et al., 1982). Other epidemiological observations have suggested that exposure to air pollutants (including the oxidant gases) is linked with increased susceptibility to infections (French et al., 1973). Although a definite correlation has not yet been demonstrated, the association of air pollution level with excessive hospitalization seems valid (Bates and Sizto, 1983).

The body has various barriers as a defence against infectious microbial agents (viruses, bacteria, fungi and parasites). Examples of physical and biochemical defences are intact skin and the barrier formed by ciliated cells and the mucous layer over them in the upper airways. In addition to these, the body is also protected by the immune system.

This system is divided into two functional entities: (1) the non-specific resistance and (2) the specific, acquired immunity. The non-specific protective mechanism is usually activated as a first line of defence and includes the uptake (phagocytosis) and killing of particles (e.g. bacteria) by polymorphonuclear leukocytes and macrophages. The specific immune system is characterised by the establishment of memory. Immunological memory means that, following a second contact with the same antigen (e.g. an infectious organism), an enhanced (secondary) response is evoked. This system is organised in central or primary lymphoid tissue, (such as bone marrow and thymus), and in peripheral or secondary lymphoid tissues (such as spleen, lymph nodes and Peyer's patches).

## Immunotoxicity testing

In order to minimise the risk of chemicals to human health, procedures have been developed to generate data on the mammalian toxicity of any chemical under investigation. Such studies include the identification of target organs of toxicity in multidose experiments lasting from 28 to 90 days. In our opinion, screening for potential immunotoxicity can best be performed within the framework of these conventional toxicology studies.

As it is practically impossible to test all chemicals for their impacts on the immune function, immunotoxicity testing for humans and rodents is preferably carried out as a tiered system (IPCS, 1986; Vos and Van Loveren, 1987). Since conventional toxicology studies are performed predominantly with rats, we chose this species as our main experimental animal.

*Tier 1* For a first tier screening, a set of general parameters of the specific and non-specific defence potential is used. General immune parameters are white blood cell counts, serum immunoglobulin concentrations of M and G class, bone marrow cellularity, and weight and histology of thymus, spleen and lymph nodes.

*Tier 2* If the screening study has provided data that suggest immunotoxicity, function studies are performed to confirm and further identify the nature of the immunotoxic effect and to determine its possible significance as a health hazard. The choice for further studies depends on the type of immune abnormality noted. Our tier 2 consists of assays covering cell-mediated immunity, humoral immunity mediated by antibodies, macrophage and natural killer cell function, and host resistance against bacterial and parasitic diseases.

*Tier 3* Further specialised experiments may become necessary to investigate the mechanism of action of the immunotoxic compound. For this purpose, an overwhelming number of tests are available that have evolved from immunology research. In particular, various in vitro assays can be of great value because they offer the opportunity to investigate the toxic action on cells of human origin.

The approach of immunotoxicity screening has been shown to be succesful in that notorious compounds, such as PCBs, dioxin and certain alkyltins, have been identified as immunotoxic environmental chemicals. The screening system described above was applied to assess the potential immunotoxicity of 18 pesticides. The most potent immunotoxic chemicals appeared to be the environmental contaminants hexachlorobenzene (HCB) and tributyltin oxide (TBTO) (see Vos et al., 1984, and Vos, 1986).

Results of the first tier screening study showed that HCB, without altering body weight, significantly increased the number of monocytes in the peripheral blood and serum IgM concentration. Moreover, HCB increased in a dose-related fashion increased the weight of spleen, and the weights of mesenteric and popliteal lymph nodes. Microscopically, the white pulp in the spleen was enlarged due to hyperplasia of follicles and marginal zones. These alterations are indications of an immune stimulatory effect of HCB. Results of the second tier function tests carried out in rats that were exposed to HCB after weaning, as well as in rats exposed pre- and postnatally, confirmed this hypothesis.

In the first tier screening study with TBTO, effects on peripheral lymphocyte and monocyte counts, and on serum IgM and IgG were already observed at a dietary level that only marginally affected body weight. The effect on thymus was predominant, already showing a significant reduction in weight at a lower level. Histopathologically the main effect was a lymphocyte depletion in the thymic cortex and in spleen and lymph nodes. From the various immune function studies, we concluded that TBTO causes a pronounced suppression of the thymus-dependent immunity and the non-specific immune system.

## Observations in wildlife populations

Most of the concern over chemical contamination effects on wildlife populations has been focused on the aquatic ecosystem. The aquatic environment has long been – and is still being – misused for the disposal of sewage, agricultural and industrial wastes. In the past decade, a growing body of literature has appeared on the effects of pollution on the health status of aquatic life. These effects have been discussed and reviewed by Dethlefsen and Tiews (1985), Malins et al. (1988), Mix and Heath (1986), Overstreet (1988), Sindermann (1983), Sindermann et al. (1980), and Vethaak (1987). These studies deal mainly with the occurrence of tumours or infectious diseases in fish. There is, however, limited information about the impact of pollution on diseases of shellfish and other invertebrates.

Figure 5.1 shows some examples of fish diseases with an infectious component that are commonly associated with pollution – such as lymphocystic infection of flatfish, and fin erosion and skin ulcer disease in various species. Since the etiology of many of these diseases is complex and multifactorial, the evidence that environmental pollution is responsible for triggering off or intensifying them remains circumstantial. Tables 5.1 and 5.2 summarise data from some surveys of neoplastic and non-neoplastic diseases in fish and in marine invertebrates, done in various places in the world, where authors have discussed their findings in relation to pollution.

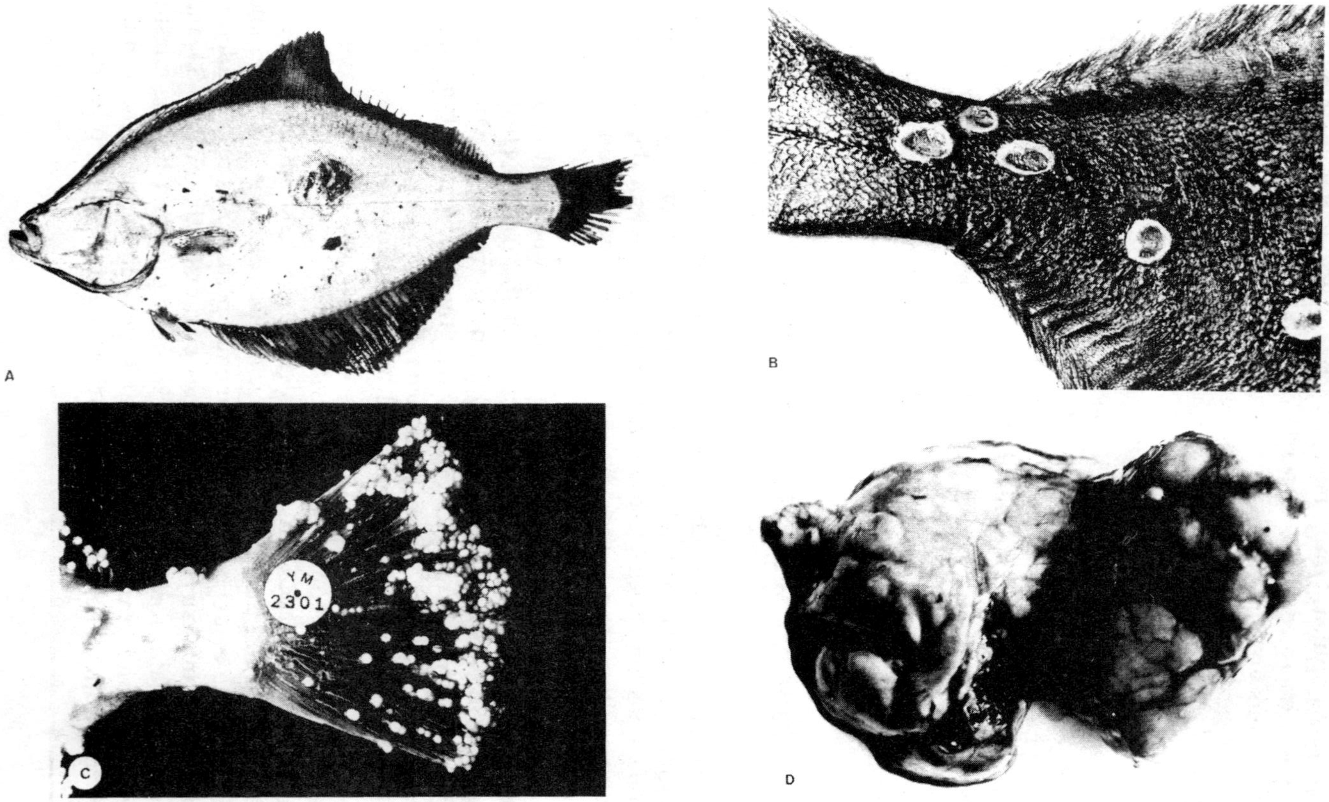


Figure 5.1 Some conditions in flounder *(Platichthys flesus)*, commonly associated with environmental pollution. (A) Fin erosion, (B) Skin ulcers, (C) Lymphocystis, (D) Liver tumours

# Assessing the toxicity of environmental chemicals for the immune systems of lower vertebrates and invertebrates

The study of the immune system of cold-blooded vertebrates and invertebrates has received considerable attention in the last decade. These comparative immunobiology studies have provided important information

**Table 5.1**
**Summary of data from some surveys of fish diseases in various sites, where authors have suggested a link with pollution.**

| Site of survey | Species involved | Disease condition | Reference |
|---|---|---|---|
| Britanny coastal waters (France) | mullet (*Mullus spp.*) | skin ulcers | Balouet, Baudin-Laurencin, 1983 |
| Dutch coastal waters | flounder (*Platichthys flesus*) | lymphocystis disease, skin ulcers, fin erosion and liver tumours | Vethaak, 1987 |
| Lower Elbe river | flounder (*Platichthys flesus*) | various liver conditions | Peters et al., 1987 |
| German Bight | dab (*Limanda limanda*) | epidermal hyperlasia/papilloma | Dethlefsen, 1984 |
| Danish coastal waters | cod (*Gadus morhua*) | skin ulcers | Jensen, 1983 |
| Baltic Sea (Sweden) | perch (*Perca fluviatilis*) | fin erosion | Lindesjöö, pers. comm. |
| New York Bight (USA) | various flatfish species | fin erosion | Murchelano and Ziskowski, 1982 |
| Puget Sound (USA) | bottom-dwellers, a.o. English sole (*Parophrys vetulus*) | liver tumours | Malins et al., 1987 |
| Black River (Ohio, USA) | brown bullhead (*Ictalurus nebulosus*) | skin and liver tumours | Baumann et al., 1987 |
| California coast (USA) | dover sole (*Microstomus pacificus*) | fin erosion | Cross, 1985 |
| Japanese waters | croaker (*Nibea mitsukurii*) | chromatophoromas | Kimura et al., 1984 |

**Table 5.2**
**Summary of data from some surveys of diseases in marine invertebrates, where authors have discussed their findings in relation to pollution.**

| Site of survey | Species involved | Disease condition | Reference |
|---|---|---|---|
| New York Bight (USA) | crustaceans | black gill disease | Sawyer et al., 1983 |
| | | black spot disease | Young and Pearcee, 1975 |
| Norwegian fjord | mussel (*Mytilus edulis*) | granulocytomas | Auffret, submitted |
| Gulf of Mexico | crustaceans | shell disease | Overstreet, 1988 |

on the evolution of the immune system. In particular they have shown that immune competence is not restricted to warm-blooded vertebrates but also occurs in cold-blooded vertebrate and invertebrate species. For example, transplantation immunity is present in earthworm and starfish, as demonstrated by the rejection of foreign skin grafts. What has also become clear is the similar organisation of different aspects of the immune response between the species, and the steadily increasing complexity and potentiality of the response – the most complex system being found in the vertebrates.

In view of these data it can be expected that chemicals which have been identified as being immunotoxic in toxicity studies with rodents also have the potential to impair the immune competence of lower species. Indeed, it has been shown under controlled laboratory conditions that environmental contaminants such as heavy metals, PCBs and certain pesticides which are immunotoxic for rodents may also interfere with the immune system of fish. *This means that an increase in infectious diseases in areas contaminated with immunotoxic chemicals could be attributed, at least in part, to the immunosuppressive properties of these compounds.*

For a proper assessment of the risk of these chemicals it is necessary to have data on target organ toxicity, i.e. on the organ or organ system in which alterations are seen using the lowest concentrations of the toxicant. Dose-response relationships are important in order to understand whether the concentrations of chemicals observed in wildlife specimens exceed the thresholds for impairment of the immune system. Hence data on immunotoxicity for rodent species – obtained for example in a tiered test system as described above – are not sufficient to evaluate the impact of environmental chemicals on the immune system of wildlife populations, although such systems can be of value in identifying candidate immunotoxic compounds.

The inclusion of immune parameters – such as morphology of the lymphoid organs or white blood cell counts – in toxicity studies with aquatic species could be used as a screening test (Zeeman and Brindley, 1981) and could be an important first step. Figure 5.2, for example, shows how thymus atrophy was observed upon microscopical investigation of TBTO-exposed guppies (Wester and Canton, 1987), which was a similar effect to that reported in the rat (Krajnc et al., 1984). It can be assumed that such immune parameters provide indications of disfunctioning of the immune system and hence can be used to predict an increased susceptibility to diseases that are under the control of the immune system. This prediction could be further tested and confirmed in a second step where the immune system is functionally assessed after controlled exposure to the test compound – an approach that is similar to the tier two testing in the rat as described above.

The aims of our future research are

(1) to validate the present immunotoxicity assessment methodology as described above in terms of toxicant-induced alterations in host resistance, and in terms of the methodologies that are used in other laboratories;

(2) to incorporate modern and more refined immunological methodologies in the immunotoxicity assessment programme.

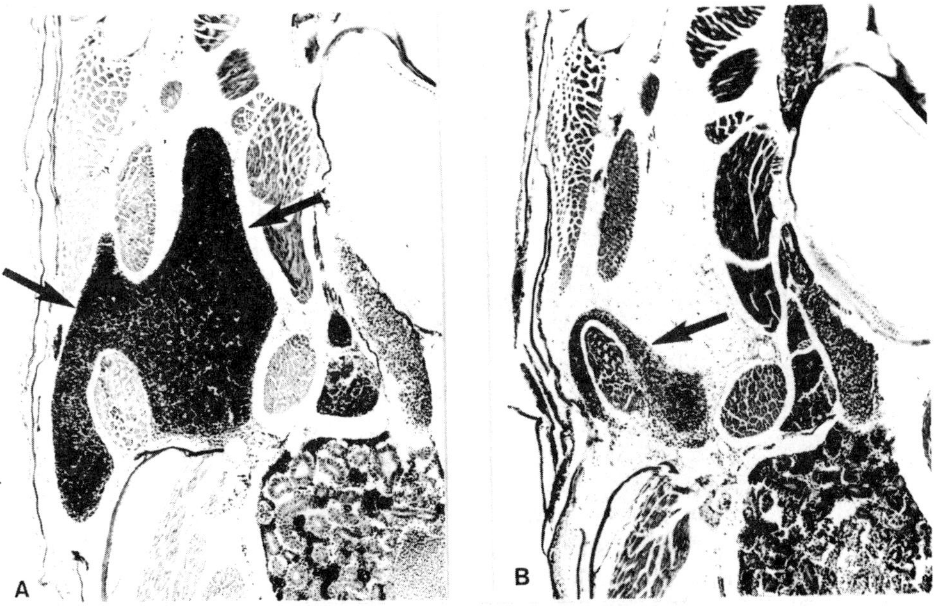


**Figure 5.2. Microscopical picture of a thymus (arrows) of (A) a control and (B) TBTO-exposed Poecilia reticulata (guppy). Severe atrophy of the thymus has occurred in (B). Hematoxylin and eosin staining, x80.**

(3) to cover all aspects of the host's immune system with the immunotoxicity assessment methodology, i.e. areas which have not yet gained much attention, such as respiratory and intestinal immunity, and also disorders such as allergy and autoimmunity, which can be a result of exposure to chemicals;

(4) to study the long-term health effects, including immunological parameters, of contaminated sediments on flatfish under controlled (semi-field) conditions;

(5) to compare these effects with those in the small fish used in the laboratory in order to validate the laboratory model for environmental toxicology.

## References


Auffret, M., 'Histopathological changes related to chemical contamination in mussels (Mytilus edulis) from field and experimental conditions', Submitted to *Marine Ecology*, Progress Series.

Bates, D.V. and Sizto, R., 'Relationship between air pollutant levels and hospital admission in Southern Ontario', *Canad. J. Publ. Health*, no. 74, 1983, pp. 117–122.

Balouet, G. and Baudin-Laurencin, F., 'Penetrating ulcers of mullet and possible relationships with petroleum', *C.I.E.M*, no. 44, 1980, pp. 1–6.

Baumann, P.C., Smith, W.D. and Pauland, W.K., 'Tumour frequencies and contaminant concentrations in brown bullheads from an industrialized river and a recreational lake', *Trans. Am. Fish. Soc.*, no. 116, 1987, pp. 79–86.

Centers for Disease Control, 'Human immunodeficiency virus (HIV) infection codes: official authorized addendum', *Morbid. Mortal. Weekly Rep.*, no. 36, 1988, pp. 1–24.

Chang, K.J., Hsieh, K.H., Tang, S.Y., Tung, T.C., and Lee, T.P., 'Immunologic evaluation of patients with polychlorinated biphenyl poisoning: evaluation of delayed-type skin hypersensitivity response and its relation to clinical studies', *J. Toxicol. Environ. Health*, no. 9, 1982, pp. 217–223.

Christensen, N.O., 'Diseases and anomalies in fish and invertebrates in Danish littoral regions which might be connected with pollution', *Rapp. P. v. Reun. Cons. int. Explor. Mer.*, no. 179, 1980, pp. 103–109.

Cross, J.N., 'Fin erosion among fishes collected near a southern California municipal wastewater outfall (1971–1982)', *Fish. Bull.*, vol. 83, no. 2, 1985, pp. 195–206.

Dethlefsen, V., 'Diseases in North Sea fishes', *Helgoländer Meeresunters*, no. 37, 1984, pp. 353–374.

Dethlefsen, V. and Tiews, K., 'Review on the effects of pollution on marine fish life and fisheries in the North Sea', *J. Appl. Ichtyol*, no. 1, 1985, pp. 97–118.

French, J.G., Lowrimore, G., Nelson, W.C., Finklea, J.F., English, T. and Herts, M., 'The effect of sulfur dioxide and suspended sulphates on averting respiratory disease', *Arch. Environ. Health* , no. 27, 1973, pp. 129–133.

IPCS, *Immunotoxicology: Development of predictive testing for determining the immunotoxic potential of chemicals*, Report of a technical review meeting, International Programme on Chemical Safety, London, 2–5 November 1986.

Jensen, N.J., 'The ulcus syndrome in cod (Gadus morhua): a review', *Rapp. P. v. Reun. Cons. int. Explor. Mer.*, no. 182, 1983, pp. 58–64.

Kimura, T., Taniguchi, N., Kumai, H., Tomita, I., Kinae, N., Yoshizaki, K., Ito, M. and Ishikawa, T., 'Correlation of epizootiological observations with experimental data: chemical induction of chromatophoromas in the croaker, *Nibea mitsukurii*', *Natl. Cancer Inst. Monogr.*, no. 65, 1984, pp. 139–54.

Krajnc, E.I., Wester, P.W., Loeber, J.G., Van Leeuwen, F.X.R., Vos, J.G., Vaessen, H.A.M.G. and Van Der Heijden, C.A., 'Toxicity of bis(tri-n-butyltin)oxide in the rat, I, Short-term effects on general parameters and on the endocrine and lymphoid system', *Toxicol. Appl. Pharmacol.*, no. 75, 1984, pp. 363–86.

Malins, D.C., McCain, B.B., Meyers, M.S., Brown, D.W., Krahn, M.M., Roubal, W.T., Schiewe, M.H., Landahl, J.T. and Chan, S.L., 'Field and laboratory studies of the etiology of liver neoplasms in marine fish from Puget Sound', *Environm. Health Perspect.*, no. 71, 1987, pp. 5–16.

Malins, D.C., McCain, B.B., Landahl, J.T., Myers, M.S., Krahn, M.M., Brown, D.W., Chan, S.L. and Roubal, W.T., 'Neoplastic and other diseases in fish in relation to toxic chemicals: an overview', *Aquat. Toxicol.*, no. 11, 1988, pp. 43–67.

Mix, M.C., 'Shellfish diseases in relation to toxic chemicals', *Aquat. Toxicol.*, no. 11, 1988, pp. 29–42.

Mix, M.C. and Heath, G.W., 'Cancerous diseases in aquatic animals and their association with environmental pollutants: a critical literature review', *Mar. Environm. Res.*, vol. 20, no. 1–2, 1986, pp. 1–141.

Murchelano, R.A. and Ziskowski, J., 'Fin rot diseases in the New York Bight (1973–1977)', in Mayer, G.F., (ed.) *Ecological stress and the New York Bight: Science and Management*, Estuary Research Foundation Columbia, S.C., 1982, pp. 347–358.

Overstreet, R.M., 'Aquatic pollution problems, Southeastern U.S. coasts: histopathological indicators', *Aquat. Toxicol.*, no. 11, 1988, pp. 213–239.

Penn, I., 'The neoplastic consequence of immunosuppression', in Berlin, A., et al. (eds.) *Immunotoxicology*, Martinus Nijhoff Publishers, Dordrecht, 1987, pp. 69–82.

Peters, N., Köhler, A. and Krantz, H., 'Liver pathology in fishes from the lower Elbe as a consequence of pollution', *Dis. Aquat. Org.*, no. 2, 1987, pp. 87–97.

Sawyer, T.K., Lewis, E.J., Galasso, M., Bodammer, S., Ziskowski, J., Lear, D., O'Malley, M. and Smith, S., 'Black gill conditions in the rock crab, *Cancer irroratus*, as indicators of ocean dumping in Atlantic coastal waters of the United States', *Rapp. P.-v. Reun. Cons. int. Explor. Mer.*, no. 182, 1983, pp. 91–95.

Sindermann, C.J., 'An examination of some relationships between pollutants and disease', *Rapp. P.-v. Reun. Cons. int. Explor. Mer.*, no. 182, 1983, pp. 37–43.

Sindermann, C.J., Bang, F.B., Christensen, N.O., Dethlefsen, V., Harshbarger, J.C., Mitchell, J.R. and Mulcahy, M.F., 'The role and value of pathobiology in pollution effects monitoring programs', *Rapp. P.-v. Reun. Cons. int. Explor. Mer.*, no. 179, 1980, pp. 135–151.

Vethaak, A.D., 'Fish diseases, signals for a diseased environment?', Proceedings of the 2nd North Sea Seminar '86, Rotterdam, 1–3 Oct., in Peet, G. (ed.), *Reasons for concern*, vol. 2, Werkgroep Noordzee, Amsterdam, 1987, pp. 41–61.

Vos, J.G., 'Immunotoxicity of hexachlorobenzene', in 'Hexachlorobenzene', in Morris, C.R. and Cabral, J.R.P., (eds.), *Proceedings of an International Symposium* , IARC, Lyon, 1986, pp. 347–356.

Vos, J.G. and Van Loveren, H., 'Immunotoxicity testing in the rat', in Burger, E.J., et al. (eds.), *Environmental Chemical Exposures and Immune System Integrity, Adv. in Mod. Environm. Toxicol.*, vol.13, Princeton Scient. Publ. Co., 1987, pp. 167–180.

Vos, J.G., De Klerk, A., Krajnc, E.I., Kruizinga, W., Van Ommen, B. and Rozing, J., 'Toxicity of bis(tri-n-butyltin)oxide in the rat, II, Suppression of thymus-dependent immune responses and of parameters of non-specific resistance after short-term exposure', *Toxicol. Appl. Pharmacol.*, no. 75, 1984, pp. 387–408.

Wester, P.W. and Canton, J.H., 'Histopathological study of *Pœcilia reticulata* (guppy) after long-term exposure to bis(tri-n-butyltin)oxide (TBTO) and di-n-butyltindichloride (DBTC)', *Aquat. Toxiol.*, no. 10, 1987, pp. 143–165.

Young, J.S. and Pearcee, J.B., 'Shell disease in crabs and lobsters from New York bight', *Mar. Poll. Bull.*, no. 6, 1975, pp. 101–105.

Zeeman, M.G. and Brindley, W.A., 'Effects of toxic agents upon fish immune systems: a review', in Sharma, R.P. (ed.), *Immunologic Considerations in Toxicology*, vol. II, CRC Press Inc., Boca Raton, Fla., 1981, pp. 1–60.

Chapter 6

# Pollution and forest die-back

by R.A. Impens, E. Laitat and J. Fagot

Forest die-back is the most obvious, but also the most complex, effect of air pollution on terrestrial ecosystems.

The die-back of main forest tree species[1], described initially in the Bohemian Mountains in Czechoslovakia, is now reported in much of the northern hemisphere, from the Appalachians in North America to Eastern Europe. The symptoms of this die-back are so variable, and a characteristic description of them so difficult to give, that it can be asked whether we are not witnessing several different diseases.

The phenomenon of die-back is worrying both the authorities and the public by its extension, its evolution, and the number and economic and ecological importance of the species concerned. This worry is all the deeper because no single theory or hypothesis among the many put forward to explain die-back can be held to be certain today.

From the forests of Central Europe, the damage spread progressively to the west. In the Federal Republic of Germany (FRG), the first areas to be hit were not the ones with a huge industrial concentration, such as the Ruhr or the Saar, but rather medium altitude areas (600 to 900m). The forests of the Ardennes, both in Belgium and in the Grand Duchy of Luxemburg, were

---

1 Picea abies (L) Kirst, Abies (Mill) sp., Fagus sylvatica L.

also hit. The symptoms of the disease were first noticed and identified on spruces and firs during the summer of 1982 in areas bordering the FRG.

The economy of these affected areas relies largely on forestry. The characteristics of these plateaux, with an elevation of 500m and above, are oligotrophic soils, a cold climate, a long period of snow and frequent fogs. The main species are spruces, with beeches more to the south.

In what follows, we shall first try to define die-back, according to Manion, then describe the symptoms of the multi-factor physiological disease, and finally look at probable hypotheses based on work done on the problem in forest research stations.

## What is forest die-back?

In his book *Tree disease concepts*, Manion (1981) tries to explain die-back as an interaction of three main factors: predisposition, contribution and incitement.

***Predisposition.*** This can be ascribed to:

- *The species and its genetic potential.* This factor seems irrelevant: resinous trees are affected the first, but many deciduous species are also damaged consequently.
- *The type of soil.* Edaphic properties and water retention seem to play a secondary role in the process. All types of soil are encountered in the damaged areas and they do not seem to play any significant role.
- *The methods of sylviculture.* These seem to have little effect: many tree species, and not only resinous ones, are being damaged, both in and out of their natural dispersion area, in natural and managed forest, with populations of the same or differing ages, and using mixed or pure cultivation methods.

***Contribution factors.*** These include biotic diseases, caused by parasitical fungi, viruses, bacterial attacks or animal predators.

***Incitement factors.*** These seem to be the most important, and climate and atmospheric pollution are foremost among them.

### *Climate*

Macro- and micro-variations of climate in the areas under study do not prevent or fundamentally modify the appearence of symptoms. The drought of 1976, often alleged to be the cause of the present die-back, actually came after the first descriptions of the disease in fir trees. To some extent, extremes in climate may worsen the lack of vigour of the decaying trees: as they are more sensitive to temperature and lack of water, they will die more readily under such circumstances.

*Atmospheric pollution*

Many air pollutants are emitted in the northern hemisphere. Some of them, like sulphur dioxide and fluorine compounds, have a direct noxious influence on tree health whenever their concentration crosses a tolerance threshold. However this condition is rarely met in European forests, except in the case of industrial accidents or when adverse meteorological conditions prevent the dispersion of pollutants for some time.

Other pollutants have phytotoxic effects resulting from chemical reactions in the air, such as ozone and other photochemical oxidants,which are produced by reactions between nitrogen oxides and hydrocarbons emitted notably by internal combustion engines.

## Symptoms of die-back

The general characteristics of forest die-back are an early falling of the leaves and a discolouration of the needles, turning yellow and brown (Schutt, 1981). In studies we have carried out in the Ardennes on resinous trees, the syndrome is differentiated according to age.

In plantations less than forty years old, some trees, or even some branches, turn irregularly yellow, then the terminal shoots become brown as early as September. The yellowing is very apparent on the upper face of the branches, especially in trees at the edge of the forest. Apical chlorosis (destruction of chlorophylls) is followed by a browning, starting in the oldest needles by mid-August, and by a die-back of some branches by the beginning of autumn (Impens et al., 1985).

In plantations of more than forty years:

- punctual, or dotted, necroses develop on needles older than one year, even on apparently healthy trees;
- the pyramidal shape can occasionally be modified;
- there is a variable clearing of branches, called 'window' starting from the inside of the crown;
- supplementary buds develop;
- second order hanging branches, sometimes stripped of their needles, are irregularly spread in the crown;
- branches become irregularly yellow.

In beech forests, the die-back begins around the crown, where long shoots with few leaves start growing. The foliage of the crown is less dense, and these sparse leaves turn prematurely yellow. These discoloured leaves are also smaller. A growing number of boughs and twigs are leafless or dry.

## Hypotheses about die-back

1. *Acidification of forest ecosystems* (Ulrich et al., 1979). Sulfate and proton fall-out, as recorded in the Solling, Hals and Harz, (south of Hannover, FRG), induce an acidification of the soil which liberates phytotoxic aluminium. This hypothesis, the oldest, called 'acid rain', is no longer a convincing explanation.

2. *Interaction of climate, parasites, and air pollution* (Rehfuess, 1985). supplemented by the influence of sylviculture methods (Cramer, 1984).

3. *Nitrogen deposits.* Pollution by nitrogen oxides ($NO_x$), due mainly to road traffic but also to ammonia emissions from intensive stock farming, is on the increase. Deposits of these compounds (40 to 60 kg nitrogen per hectare) disturb the trees' nutrition cycle. Nitrogen compounds are directly assimilated by trees, making for a high amino-acid and amide content in leaves). Roots absorb preferentially $NH_4^+$ and do so on acid soils by exchanging it for protons. These, in turn, acidify the soil and increase the mobility and leaching of positive $Mg^{++}$, $Ca^{++}$ and $K^+$ ions. Acidification, a deficiency in some major ions and a decreased use of available nitrogen are the results.

This imbalance is made even worse by the damage to and disappearence of mycorrhizes (symbiosis between a mushroom's mycelium and plant roots). These are important in safeguarding the healthy condition of trees, by their action at the root/soil interface. Reducing the extent of mycorrhization means a decrease in the efficiency of the tree's radicular system in the absorption of water and minerals, and therefore a modification of its metabolism and an increased sensitivity to drought and secondary infections.

The reduction of the mycorrhize-forming mycoflora could be due to an increase of the amount of nitrogen in soils (Meyer, 1985), but could also result from the characteristic weakening of the foliage linked to die-back, which would provide fewer glucidic metabolites to the fungi. This reduction, then, would be both an effect and a cause of forest die-back. Recent monitoring in affected areas has shown that sizeable changes in this mycoflora have taken place (Guillitte, 1987).

4. *Ozone.* The presence of photochemical compounds, including ozone (produced in particular in reaction with $NO_x$, together with relatively poor soils and acidic fog, could explain the symptoms and damage observed (Prinz et al., 1982). High ozone concentrations are not uncommon in the Ardennes. Ozone increases cell membrane permeability in resinous needles, thus inducing an uncontrolled ion loss by leaching in rain or fog. Possible effects on stomata aperture regulation would also increase water loss and contribute to the tree's hydric imbalance. This type of damage increases in sunny weather on poor soils. Chronic exposure to ozone brings about a

decrease in soluble sugars and is associated with a reduction in root growth – with its consequences on mycorrhization.

## Conclusions

Forest die-back is a new disease caused by several factors, each of which contributes to weakening the trees.

Initially, so-called 'acid rain' was considered responsible for the damage. But further analyses and studies carried out in the European Community and the United States now point rather to air pollutants such as $NO_x$, ozone and other photochemicals as the cause.

The decrease in sulphur dioxide emissions observed in the last ten years has been offset by increasing emissions of $NO_x$ and hydrocarbons generating oxidisers, such as ozone and photochemical smog. Without neglecting the influence of sulphur dioxide and sulphate deposits, it would seem that the joint effect of nitrogen compound deposits and ozone might account for the damage we have witnessed in recent years over vast forest areas.

On poor soils, which are usually reserved for forestry, and in periods of intense sunlight, all the conditions are met for leaf cells to be attacked: ion and water losses, damage to chlorophyll and intracellular structures, etc. The results are water supply imbalance, cation loss, reduction of photosynthesis, modifications in mycorrhize formation around roots, and a general weakening of the tree, which then becomes more sensitive to climatic change and less resistant to its natural parasites.

Forest die-back has given rise to numerous and complex research programmes in most countries where it occurs. It has made us aware of the gaps in our knowledge of tree physiology and particularly of tree metabolism. The difficulty of carrying out experiments on trees, because of their longevity and the sheer complexity of pollution and climatic factors, must make us think twice about claiming to understand the mechanisms of die-back. Only concerted, long-term action at European level, bringing together field work and laboratory experiments, might give us any hope of discovering the causes of this phenomenon. Solutions must, in any event, include a drastic reduction in pollutant emissions. The authorities of all European countries concerned will have to act together to achieve this.

# References


Cramer, H.H., 'Über die Dispositionen Mittel-europäischer Forsten für Waldschäden', *Pflanzenschutz-Nachrichten Bayer*, no. 37(2), 1984, pp. 97–207.

Guillitte, O., 'Observations mycologiques et "pluies acides" en Belgique', *Mém. Soc. Roy. Bot. Belg.*, no. 9, 1987, pp. 67–8.

Impens, R., Delcarte, E., Robert, M.J. and Tilman, J., 'Bilan de l'exploitation d'un réseau de plantes indicatrices de la pollution atmosphérique', *C.R. Symp. Vle Congrès mondial pour la Qualité de l'Air*, Paris, May 1985, no. 2, pp. 541–547.

Impens, R., Laitat, E., Derouane, A., Meurrens, A. and Delcarte, E., 'Le réseau de surveillance du dépérissement des forêts belges', *Pollution atmosphérique*, Jan.–March 1985, pp. 16–23.

Laitat, E. and Fagot, J., 'Etude du dépérissement forestier en Belgique. Premier bilan d'une année de récolte des précipitations à la station pilote de Vielsalm', Commission des Communautés Européennes: *Pollution de l'air et écosystèmes*, proceedings of an international conference held in Grenoble, France, 18–22 May 1987, pp. 554–559.

Manion, P.D., *Tree disease concepts*, Prentice Hall, 1981.

Meyer, F.H., 'Root and mycorrhiza development in declining forests', *Indirect effects of air pollution on forest trees*, Proceedings of COST Workshop, Julich (FRG), 5–6 Dec. 1985., pp. 139–151.

Prinz, B., Krause, G. and Stratmann H., 'Waldschäden in der Bundesrepublik Deutschland', *LIS Berichte*, no. 28, 1982, p. 148.

Rehfuess, K.E., 'Maladies de la forêt et pollution de l'air', *Parasitica*, no. 41 (3), 1985, pp. 127–34.

Schutt, P., 'Das Krankheitsbild, verschiedene Baumarte, gleiche Symptome', *Bild der Wissenschaft*, no. 12, 1981, pp. 86–101.

Ulrich, B., Mayer, B. and Khanna, P.K., 'Deposition von Luftverunreinigungen und ihre Auswirkungen im Waldökosystem in Solling', *Schriften Forstl., Fak. Univ. Göttingen u. Hieders Forstl. Versuchsanstalt*, 1979.

Chapter 7

# Environment and skin ageing

by Micheline Song

Skin ageing is a complex phenomenon whose fundamental mechanisms are not known, but in which time, genetic and environmental factors all play an important part.

A major influence on cell functioning is time but others factors may strengthen it: the environment, the use of drugs, internal metabolic or hormonal factors and external factors such as actinic radiation.[1] When parts of the skin, such as the face or hands, are exposed to light, natural ageing is significantly intensified. Genetic factors have a role too, and in some hereditary diseases the skin of a young child can show disorders similar to those of an old person.

Some theories have been put forward to explain certain aspects of ageing.

- The *theory of the programme* considers that cells have a limited number of possible multiplications, and that at the end of the programme growth stops and the cells die.
- The *theory of errors* holds that through successive cell divisions errors in the copying of genetic material can occur, with the action of aggressive endogenic or exogenic factors perhaps changing the DNA restoring mechanisms.

---

1 Radiation which produces chemical changes.

- The *control theory* sees cell multiplication control being provided by growth factors and hormones. During the ageing process there is a reduction of endocrine secretions and of their receptors on membranes.

Skin modifications associated with ageing vary from one place to another. They are most obvious in the uncovered parts of the skin often exposed to sunlight in patients of white race, so the role of sunlight in skin ageing has been suspected for a long time. And it has been demonstrated that keratinocytes from a skin exposed to the sun have a shorter lifespan in culture than those from a protected skin.

However, the role played by each of the types of radiation reaching the earth's surface is not well known yet. A and B ultra-violet probably play the most important part, but visible light and infra-red could also be active. The degree of modification depends, on the one hand, on the duration and the intensity of exposure (altitude, latitude, season, hour, weather, ground reflection) and, on the other hand, on the protection and recovery mechanisms of the organism (thickness of the horny layer, melanin pigmentation, integrity of the DNA restoring system).

The protective role of the *stratum corneum* against UV radiation is linked to its melanin content: that of a black skin lets through less than fifty per centof the light absorbed by a white skin. And the organism takes advantage of both the pigmentation and the thickness of the epidermis to prevent UV ray penetration. One of the first results of radiation is in fact the thickening of the epidermis and pigmentation. This screening function takes place for all wavelengths since infra-red rays are also absorbed by the water content of the *stratum corneum.*

In the long term, solar radiation induces skin modifications in both the epidermis and the dermis. In the epidermis, keratinocytes become more densely packed, and in the basal layer some modification of cell proliferation in dividing cells takes place, which in turn may be responsible for benign or malignant tumours (keratoses, basocellular and spinocellular epitheliomas).

In the pigment system, both the activity and the amount of melanin are reduced through the effect of solar radiation. The role of melanin is important, as it is both a solar filter and a captor of the free radicals liberated by UV rays. Its alteration will lead to the accumulation of toxic substances and thus favour neoplasic modifications. In the exposed areas, a heterogeneous pigmentation will progressively appear in both hyperpigmented and unpigmented areas.

## Changes to the dermis

The dermis is the compartment where age-linked and environment-linked modifications are the most obvious. The number and the activity of cells is reduced and actinic radiation penetrating the dermis greatly modifies the fibres (collagen fibres of the reticulate dermis disappear almost completely, while elastic fibres are modified) and an interfibrillary substance appears. Morphological alterations of blood vessel walls may be seen in the exposed areas. The consequence is a reduced intake of metabolites, but also a local accumulation of waste. The skin is pale, scars heal more slowly, and there are problems of thermoregulation.

In addition, free radicals produced by ionising radiation alter various macromolecules and senile atrophy results from a decreasing synthesis of macromolecules in the conjunctive tissue, without a proportionate reduction in catabolism. The result of such modifications is a thin and fragile skin.

## The principal risk factors

An epidemiological study published in the United States in 1988[2], about the effects of sun radiation on the skin, shows that the main risk factors are: amount of UV, age, male gender, light eye colour, white race. The main effects are:

- irregular pigmentation
- keratosis, lentiginosis
- malignancies: basocellular and spinocellular epitheliomas (proliferative disorders)
- lesions of the mouth mucous membranes, of the tongue and of the palate.

Malignant melanomas were not listed in this study, but epidemiological studies have shown that such cancers are found on skin areas exposed to light.

Wind and moisture seem unable to induce skin alterations linked to ageing, but they might compound the effect of UV.

As for air pollution, some chemicals could act directly on the skin, such as arsenic or tar. Others act indirectly by reducing the ozone layer, a natural screen against UV. The risks of exposure to UV radiation could increase in the future, due to the partial depletion of the ozone layer. The increase in skin cancer frequency has been estimated at four per cent for every one per cent decrease of the layer, and this does not take account of melanic tumours.

Finally, some recent studies on hairless mice have shown that low-dose, sub-erythemateous irradiation with a xenon lamp (emitting both UV-A and

2 Engel, A., Johnson, M.L. and Haynes, S., 'Health effects of sunlight exposure in the United States', *Arch. Dermatol.*, vol. 124, 1988, pp. 72–79.

UV-B) significantly worsens skin ageing, while natural ageing during the same time (two years) has little effect. Thus, even in low doses, sunlight is an important factor in the skin ageing process.

It has now been shown that preventive action can be taken against the worsening of natural ageing through exposure to sunlight. Its purpose is to reduce the cumulative dose for radiation of all kinds. Skin protection by screening of the sun's rays should not be kept only for cases of occasional intense radiation, but should be practised permanently on those areas of the skin most exposed to damage. Moreover, it is hoped that UV-induced modifications might be treated by a local use of retinoids (vitamin A acid).

Thus, skin ageing is the result of many factors: genetic, metabolic, internal and environmental. And the development of skin cancers is now considered with certainty to be the consequence of a chronic exposure to ultra-violet rays.

Chapter 8

# Electromagnetic pollution of the environment

by Wolfgang Volkrodt

People have known about electromagnetic waves for about a century. It was not until after World War II, however, that we started to use them extensively in technical applications. Over the last thirty years, transmission density has doubled every four years or so, which means that electromagnetic pollution has gone up around 100 times. In addition, the wavelengths used are getting shorter; we have now entered the microwave era where we are dealing with minuscule dimensions. Microwaves are used, for example, in air traffic control (5, 10 and 23 cm) and directional transmitters (1.5–20 cm).

Microwaves then, are nothing new. Microwaves measuring between approximately 1 cm and several metres reach the planet's surface through the 'window' in the radiological protection belt of the earth's atmosphere. The shorter the waves, the more energy they produce. At $10^{-10}$ mW/cm$^2$ (milliwatt/square centimetre), performance capacity is low, but biological systems nevertheless use microwave energy to supplement light to meet their energy needs. For instance, we speak in microwave parlance when measuring leaf ribs and pine needles. If leaf ribs were really just 'plumbing' – tubes to transport moisture – they would be constructed in a different way.

## Microwaves: a grave risk

Microwaves cause cell destruction and are inimical to life, both from thermal effects on cell tissue and by interfering with normal cell processes, so they need to be carefully dosed for safety, like X-rays or gamma rays. Today, trees and other biological systems are being subjected to microwave radiation several billion times higher than naturally ordained.

In its own way, a tree is like a factory producing wood. Radar equipment or directional senders can interfere and put the 'factory' out of commission, and the tree does not know how to protect or cure itself. Small wonder that their 'biological antennae' burn out.

The Federal Republic of Germany has laid down maximum levels for artificial microwaves which only take account of the thermal effect on humans within the defined acceptable range of exposure.[1] This effectively means accepting exposure to radiation which is several billion times higher than that received from natural, cosmic sources. No account has been taken of non-thermal effects, to our deadly peril.

## Biological information systems: how do they work?

We need to know more about how biological information systems work to explain the extent of the damage done by microwaves.

All individual life functions according to a blueprint locked into the DNA molecules of the cell nucleus. Life cannot be sustained when the DNA information is lost or when it can no longer be copied and transmitted. The production of DNA copies is not a matter of chance: outside triggers are needed. Even a man-made megabit-chip will not release 'locked' information until it is told to do so. Biological instructions to copy DNA are usually triggered by chemically unstable molecules or by changing electromagnetic fields. In the process of replicating itself, the DNA molecule rotates every 1/1,000 of a second whereby electrical charges are transferred between the affected sequences of molecules. These charge transfers are necessarily coupled with electromagnetic waves. Currently, it is believed that the frequency lies in the range of micro-infrared wave lengths, depending on the speed of the replication.

In addition to the life-sustaining processes in the multiplication and distribution of DNA, living systems also exchange information in other ways:

- the exchange between individual cells or cell groups (e.g. the immune system);

---

1 Regulation DIN VDE 0848/2.

- the reciprocal exchange between cooperating organs (e.g. food ingestion and digestion);
- the nerve paths to the 'main computer' (neurons and transmitter signals to the brain where they become consciousness – e.g. sensual perception);
- the exchange between members of the same species (in humans this mostly takes the form of speech; in trees this might be UV light signals).

The signal frequency used will determine how vigorously these processes take place. In living creatures using magnetic field sensors to find their way through the earth's magnetic field, information exchange will be slow. But a stumble in a human being will provoke lightning exchange to prevent bones being broken. No computer can yet compete with nature in this respect.

All biological information systems use electromagnetic fields and waves in frequencies ranging from zero hertz (in electromagnetic field orientation) to 25 Hz (the sleeping brain) to gigahertz microwaves to the very high frequencies of light. Light is important not only to plants for photosynthesis, but to all living creatures because it regulates biological rhythms. Biological systems, however, have no use for the shortest wavelengths, such as X-rays or gamma-rays, because of their ionizing and cell destructive effects.

We now understand a little better how information is transmitted through the human nervous system. But only recently did we find out that plants have nervous systems that are similar to those of human beings. Not only are plants able to move, they even have feelings. A Heidelberg University team has discovered chemically unstable signalling materials which are to plants what neuro-transmitters are to the human brain. Known as 'turgorines', they regulate certain plant functions such as water distribution and the preparation for 'sleep' – the drooping or curling up of leaves at sundown.

Biological information and regulatory systems are surprisingly quiet performers. They emit no more than a thermo-molecular murmur, proportionately somewhat like the wind rustling through the forest. A 'word' spoken at less than that murmur will not be heard. All living species need such screening of extraneous noise. People would fall ill in body and mind if they constantly received impressions from the functioning of other biological systems. Take the rumbling of a hungry stomach as an example. A tree is no different.

Information transmission at this low noise level presupposes a range of special physical effects. In 1982, scientists suggested that superconductors and the Josephson Effect play a key role in life processes. Recent experiments with high-conductor organic molecular chains at relatively high temperatures tend to bear this out. The Josephson Effect enables a pair of electrons to 'bore through' the barrier of, for instance, a cell membrane.

Josephson elements may function as detectors, generators, mixers and reinforcers, so that they are ideal links in the information chain.

While biological research has demonstrated the sensitivity of living systems to thermal noise, no such reactions have been measured at higher power densities in systems using Josephson effects. This lack of reaction could help to explain certain widespread errors in our thinking. Research into forest pollution for example has, of course, included work on the effects of microwaves on plant cells. The radiation values used were close to technically acceptable maximum levels and no evidence of damage was ever found. The researchers concluded that at lower radiation levels, such as those used in directional transmitters, microwaves could therefore not possibly do any harm (Bernhardt et al., 1983).

While the theory of biological information systems and the question of whether or not they make use of cosmic microwave radiation is still a matter of speculation, there is now clear evidence that man-made microwaves are harmful after all. Man-made microwaves are different from cosmic 'white noise' not only because of official sanction of a billion times the cosmic radiation intensity, but also because of their precise transmission frequencies, the polarization of the waves, and modulated digital and analogous signals. These special features make them highly suspect as producing typical interference with biological information systems. We also know that such 'scramblers' can make it impossible to understand important information – witness the whines and other noises which for decades have made gibberish of Western radio broadcasts to the Soviet Union.

## Is microwave pollution killing our forests?

We can differentiate between 'traditional' and 'modern' forms of forest pollution. Traditional forms of pollution, for example atmospheric pollution following volcanic eruptions and industrial processes, have been around for a long time. 'Modern' forest pollution, on the other hand, may occur in otherwise clean environments. In my opinion, a case in point is northern Canada, where the radar installations set up to monitor Soviet air movements are wreaking widespread havoc in the forests. Similar 'radar damage' is, I believe, evident in the oak forests north of Vienna, and in the FRG in the vicinity of the Wasserkuppe mountain and near major airports such as Frankfurt am Main. There is evidence that the military and radar equipment manufacturers have known of this for years, but have kept silent for fear of massive compensation payments to forest owners.[2]

---

2 Personal contacts with the German military by the author.

Meanwhile, the radio link systems, which have taken over from cable to keep us abreast of the news, have burnt such a swathe through our forests that even laymen can see what is happening. Trees die like flies in a straight line running between the transmitters. Fourteen instances of damage from transmitters under the control of the Federal Postal Authority and twenty instances of military transmitter damage were registered in the Hunsrück, FRG region alone.

The German Postal Authority knows about the fatal damage done to our forests by directional radio. It has decided to refuse to supply information about the location and direction of these transmitters on the grounds that this is privileged information. Nature protection organisations are now searching for the country's 'fleet' of directional transmitters and the corresponding paths of destruction. In a letter dated March 30, 1987 the Ministry of Telecommunications asked the Ministry of Environment, Nature Protection and Nuclear Safety to study the following question: 'How do the performance, frequency, modulation and pulse rates of modulated microwave fields affect radiated tissue and plant cells?' [3]

Furthermore, according to the media, some seventy per cent of German citizens suffer pains, thirty per cent are the victims of allergies and fifteen per cent have to put up with constant noises in the ear (tinnitus). These are mostly disorders for which there is no discernable organic cause. Something has gone wrong with the human nervous system, we say. The environment is to blame.

But I believe, much as with our forests, that such disorders are closely connected with radiation from radio and directional transmittors. We have no conclusive proof of this as yet. To find it, we need the work of interdisciplinary research teams including high frequency experts, radiation physicists, doctors and biologists.

The FRG government has calculated that forest die-back is costing the country 5.5–8.8 billion Deutschmarks (DM) a year (some US$ 3–5 billion). By the year 2010, we shall not only have sustained a financial loss of over DM 200 billion, our forests and no doubt large numbers of people will likewise have been irreversibly damaged.

## Putting an end to microwave technology

But the future looks brighter. We can easily get rid of microwave technology. The FRG and industries have agreed that by the year 2010, communications transmissions will be achieved through a national network

3 Letter from the Federal Minister for Post and Communications to the Petitions Committee of the Federal Parliament (Bundestag) of 30 March 1987.

of modulated fibre optic conductor cables. After that the surfeit of microwave transmitters, in particular directional transmitters, will no longer be necessary. Military radar installations need to be dismantled just as missiles do. Until they are, testing should be at greater intervals and for shorter periods, just as is the case for civil air-raid sirens.

As we switch to modulated fibre optic cables, we will put an end to the interference with biological antenna currently caused by massive microwave radiation, and so steadily prevent more and more environmental damage.

We need to pull ourselves together and work flat out to speed up the transition from microwave technology to fibre optic technology. We are waging war on environmental damage and we must win the battle against the consequences of inexcusable technical shortsightedness.

## References


Baranski, S., Czerski, P., *Biological effects of microwaves,* Dowden, Hutchinson & Ross, Stroudsburg (Pa.), 1976.

Bernhardt, J.H., 'Biologisch-technische Grundlagen der Schutzbestimmungen für hochfrequente elektromagnetische Felder', in G. Newi (ed.), *Biologische Wirkungen elektrischer, magnetischer und elektromagnetischer Felder,* Expert, Grafenau, 1983.

Bernhardt, J.H., Dahme, M. and Raabe, F.K., *Gefährdung von Personen durch electromagnetische Felder,* Reimer, Berlin, 1983.

Calle, E.E., et al., 'Leukaemia in occupational groups with presumed exposure to electrical and magnetic fields', *The New England Journal of Medicine,* vol. 313, no. 23, 1985, pp. 1476–7.

Frucht, A.H., et al., *Die Wirkung hochfrequenter elektromagnetischer Felder auf den Menschen,* Institut zur Erforschung elektrischer Unfälle der Berufsgenossenschaft der Feinmechanik und Elektrotechnik, Cologne, 1984.

*Microwave News,* 'A Report on Non-Ionizing Radiation', vol. 6, no. 2, 1986.

NCRP-Report No. 86, *Biological effects and exposure criteria for radio-frequency electromagnetic fields,* NCRP, Bethesda (Md.), 1986.

Pearce, N.E., et al., 'Leukaemia in electrical workers in New Zealand', *Lancet,* no. 1, 1985, pp. 811–12.

Roberts, N.J., et al., 'Epidemiological Studies of Human Exposures to Radiofrequency Radiation', *Int. Arch. Occup. Environ. Health,* vol. 56, 1985, pp. 169–78.

Chapter 9

# Electromagnetic and ideological pollution of the brain

by José M.R. Delgado

Our group has been investigating the sources, consequences, prevention and treatment of two main aspects of pollution which in general have been neglected: a) *Biological Effects* determined by electromagnetic radiation; and b) *Neuronal Modifications* determined by cultural indoctrination.

Life has evolved under the influence of two omnipresent forces, gravity and electromagnetic interactions, and it is assumed that both play significant roles in biological activities.

We should remember that most organisms are structured by chemical dipoles, including amino acids which have both negatively charged carboxilic groups and positively charged aminic groups. It should be expected that these electrically charged particles can be modified by the application of electromagnetic fields (EMF).

The biological importance of EMF has been well substantiated in numerous publications and meetings, but our understanding about mechanisms of action is still poor. This knowledge is essential for possible beneficial effects, for adequate preventive measures and for legislation to control private and public use of electricity.

Unfortunately, the modern proliferation of electric plants, high power lines, and electrically mechanised homes are sources of artificial magnetic fields which may influence biological activities. A summary of legal standards has been published by Romero-Sierra (1981) and additional information prepared by the United Nations may be found in *Health Physics* (1984). According to these recommendations, the occupational exposure to frequencies of 10 Mhz - 300 GHz should be below 0.4 W/kg. These figures are modified by several variables, as reported in a previous publication (Delgado, 1984), and especially by the existence of 'windows' of particularly effective frequencies. New proposals to limit the exposure of workers have been presented in the United Kingdom,[1] in the Federal Republic of Germany[2] and in the People's Republic of China.[3]

Some of the experimental results of our group using weak, very low frequency EMF (Delgado, 1985) may be summarised as follows:

1. The orientation of free moving snails may be influenced by EMF.
2. Specific rotation of polarised light induced by 'In vitro' solutions of different amino acids is modified by EMF.
3. Synthesis of T-RNA may also be influenced by EMF.
4. Bacterial growth of Lactobacillus acidophilus may be inhibited with a dose-response effect by applying pulsed magnetic fields about 20 Gauss/26 Hz. Other micro-organisms may also be sensitive to EMF, introducing the possibility of therapeutic applications.
5. Exposure of male Drosophila for 70 hours to 16 Hz pulses magnetic fields of 3.5 mili Tesla produced a significant sex-linked recessive lethal mutation. This irreversible process may persist for generations, transmitted by the females which carry but are not affected by the lethal agent.
6. The unitary discharge of the crayfish stretch receptor may be influenced by application of pulsed EMF. This effect may be related to the opening and closing of membrane ionic channels.
7. Teratogenic effects have been produced by exposing developing chick embryos to pulsed EMF with intensities as low as 1 μT. Pulse shape and time of development are critical factors for the observed effects. The mitotic index may also be influenced by MEF.
8. Daily exposure of rats to EMF (50 Hz, 1.5 mT) for 18 hours during 10 days produced a significant decrease in blood gamma globulins without changes in alfa and beta globulins. These effects may have important immunological consequences.
9. In monkeys, central nervous system excitability has been influenced by EMF focused on the cerebellum. The use of this non-invasive methodology may have important applications for research and for therapy.

---

1 NRPB, 1982.

2 DIN 57848.

3 Han-Kui et al., 1982; see also Delgado, 1984.

10. In patients with pseudo-arthrosis or with delay in calcification, application of pulsed EMF (14 Hz, 15 Gauss), accelerated osteogenesis and bone repair.
11. Using a Hall sensor, we have demonstrated that motors with plastic covers used in many home appliances may give environmental pollution values as high as 25 Gauss, representing a serious risk. Powerful generators with good metallic shielding, such as power plant turbines, X-ray equipment, video monitors and computer rooms, gave comparatively low values of EMF pollution.

In Sweden, France, Germany and other countries, some of the companies which produce electrical energy are promoting investigations about EMF which may resolve unfounded fears about manufacturing and transmission of electricity, providing at the same time the necessary information about possible risks and therapeutical uses.

Utilisation of EMF energy represents problems and benefits for mankind requiring intelligent, ethical evaluation of results.

## Ideological pollution

Human beings may be modified in their genes, in their brains and in their hearts. This new biological reality represents a scientific and cultural revolution of powerful consequences.

As expressed by Alexis Carrel in his book *Man, the Unknown*, we cannot undertake the restoration of ourselves and our environment before having transformed our habit of thought. Carrel stated that 'As much importance should be given to feelings as to thermodynamics' and that 'The study of moral, esthetic, and religious functions would appear as indispensable as that of mathematics, physics or chemistry'. Thus mental activities should be considered as important as physiological ones.

Human destiny is escaping natural determinism, and gradually coming under the direction of our own intelligence. Already there are proposals for the engineering of the brain, and for a psychocivilised education able to create a society less robotized, with greater freedom, responsibility and happiness. This would represent a change in political and educational priorities, with less resources wasted in war efforts and more attention dedicated to individual and social welfare.

The problem is that governments and political groups usually try to develop their educational programmes shaping infantile minds with the purpose to provide continuity and give power to their own ideological, emotional and cultural systems. This is true in dictatorial regimes where intellectual dissidence is strongly repressed and it also occurs in democratic countries where powerful elements of social conformism exist.

Histological, embryological, and behavioural studies show that human beings are born with a very undeveloped brain lacking the most important mental functions. During the first weeks of post-natal life there is a very active development of neurons and connections, with the appearance of 'spines', arborisations, synapses and new neurochemical activities. In the absence of sensory inputs and information, the neurons will not develop and will remain in their infantile stage.

Personal identity and frames of reference are stored perhaps in the limbic system. In this way ideologies and experiences are materialised as anatomical and chemical traces which influence decisively most neuronal activities.

The biological structure of man is the egalitarian feature that unifies the origin, existence and destiny of all human beings. The *Biological Unity* of the human race has a functional and cultural transcendence that has been underevaluated. Struggles between Capitalist and Marxistic systems; hatred between Jews and Arabs; racial, religious and ideological hostilities, do have cultural bases but they are *Antibiological.*

Unfortunately there is a very subtle but powerful and widespread danger related to modern mass media communication technologies determining an *Ideological Pollution of the Brain:* minds and bodies are directed with objectives related to political and industrial interest. Beliefs, ideologies, ethics and behavioural patterns are inculcated within infantile minds, *Without the Knowledge or Consent* of the individuals (Delgado, 1969). Mental and physiological functions are usurped by hidden forces without concern for personal identity. A sensation of freedom may be given when in reality there is a manipulation of motivations and actions. It is essential to be aware of the many dangers caused by the *Neurobiological Pollution* and solutions must be found for the prevention and management of undesirable consequences.

Anticipatory long-term planning, avoidance of short-term crisis and specially a new and realistic education adapted to the present, and not to the past, are essential for the survival of mankind. Our ecological, and political, decisions are usually 'value-dependent' and therefore related to evolving ethics and conditions. It is, however, far preferable to propose 'value-free' decisions based on objective, scientifically tested reality, avoiding ideological bias. A value-free analysis could provide credible information to the public, thus supporting a sound governmental policy.

# References


Carrell, Alexis, *L'homme, cet inconnu*, Paris, Plon et Nourrit, 1935.

Delgado, J.M.R., *Physical Control of the Mind: Toward a Psychocivilized Society*, in Anshen, R.N. (ed.), World Perspectives Series, vol. XLI, New York, Harper and Row, 1969.

Delgado, J.M.R., 'Acciones Biológicas de Campos Electromagnéticos Hidroeléctrica Española: XXII Ciclo de Conferencias', Madrid, 1984.

Delgado, J.M.R., Leal, J., Monteagudo, J.L. and Garcia Gracia, M., Embryological Changes Induced by Weak, Extremely Low Frequency Electromagnetic Fields, *J. Anat.*, no. 134, 1982, pp. 533–51.

*Health Physics*, vol. 46, no. 4, 1984.

Romero-Sierra, C., 'Bioeffects of Electromagnetic Waves', in Bowhill, S.A. (ed.), *URSI Review of Radio Science, 1978-1980*, International Union of Radio Science, Brussels, 1981.

Chapter 10

# The model of the human operator system: a heuristic aid against modern anxiety

by Jacques Douchamps

The extensive and intensive exchange of information taking place within our technological world constitutes the main foundation of its development. It imposes, however, a type of stress which is definitely different from the kind of stress our organism was designed to cope with and has adapted to over the ages. In the midst of life, there is no longer time for philosophical questioning, nor for the complex but necessary integration of all new events into our basic personality structure.

While scientific discoveries highlight our complete interdependence with our environment, most often we continue to adopt old, inflexible attitudes and behaviour patterns for our everyday lives. The increasing scale of mental illnesses as well as the widespread use of legal and prohibited drugs are striking evidence of the unprecedented crisis in our society (Siegrist et al., 1984).

The idea has progressively emerged that the sole solution for mankind's survival is to develop further consciousness in all individuals (Douchamps and Hatayama, 1986; Ledoux, 1985). A new kind of human capable of a more complete perception and understanding of the self, and thus, of the individual's place in the world, is now considered as the next step of evolution. However, a more comprehensive awareness of one's self cannot be gained simply through pure scientific work. Any technical tool should integrate a classic experimental context with an experiential one.

The model of the Human Operator System (HOS), conceived from the essential principles of modern psychology, provides an easy, heuristic framework to help people realise the extent of their conditioning and the sources of the stress they feel. ('Heuristic' describes a system in which one discovers things for oneself.) Below we explain the Human Operator System and the concept of consciousness that one seeks when using it (Douchamps and Hatayama, 1988. The HOS model itself is described in detail in Douchamps, 1985, 1986a and 1986b.).

## The Human Operator System

The HOS Model sprang from the triune brain model (MacLean, 1985). MacLean considered that, in evolution, the primate forebrain expands along the lines of three basic patterns that may be characterised as reptilian (reticular formation), paleomammalian (limbic system) and neomammalian (neocortex), and that there exists, so to speak, a hierarchy of three-brains-in-one – in short, a 'triune' brain. In the triune model the brain is likened to an information processing system dealing with events according to tridimensional metrics. We assumed that the three cerebrotypes (the reticular formation, limbic system and neocortex) behave like three filters. Beyond the anecdotal memory content of any incoming event, they generate a three-dimensional mental workload reflecting the relevance of the event for the individual's survival (Figure 10.1).

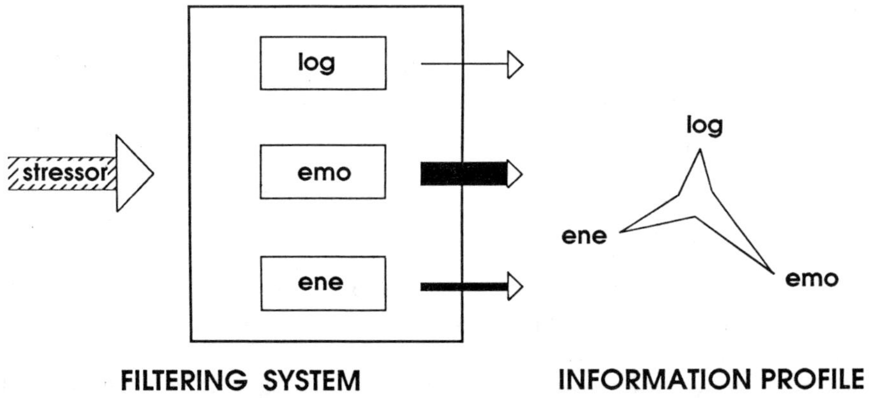


**Figure 10.1 The information profile of an incoming event is expressed as a three dimensional workload (energy/emotion/logic) elaborated by the three filters of the filtering system. The present figure describes the case of a stressor with a high emotional component.**

In this framework, behaviour related to metabolic energy (feeding, sleeping, fighting, etc.) has an important 'energetic' (ENE) workload component. Behaviour that is basically related to anguish is essentially 'emotional' (EMO); while rational thinking, whether analytic or synthetic, implies a high 'computational or logico-associative' (LOG) component. To give clear-cut examples, a marathon race is a stressful event with a main 'ENE' component; the loss of a parent is an 'emotional' (EMO) stressor; and the solving of a difficult mathematical problem is a stressor of the 'computational' (LOG) type.

In addition, the processing of any event necessitates the recall of related anecdotal memories and the use of a 'software'. Both functions have recourse to the individual's metacognitive knowledge – i.e., the whole content of memory – which is elaborated over the years as a function of the person's basic capabilities and experiences.

The simple processing of events is carried out by a myriad of small peripheral processing units. Complex processing takes place simultaneously within two parallel central units; the left one is more specialised in analytical reasoning, while the right unit is more dedicated to analogical abstractions (at least in the idealised case of an average right-handed, western subject, as shown in Figure 10.2).

Both central processing units are monitored by their own supervisory systems, each of which encompasses a regulator and a 'conscioustiser'. As shown in Figure 10.2, the regulator generates awareness and the 'conscioustiser' generates consciousness. The various levels of awareness and consciousness engendered depend on the complexity of the information processing taking place in the central units. The resulting extent of awareness – which is experienced as an 'inner', pre-verbal sensation – is the integrated outcome of both left and right processes controlled by the regulator(s). Similarly, consciousness can result from both left and right side chains of processing and emerges when a chain uses a highly complex piece of software involving the conscioustiser(s). In sum, awareness corresponds to a pre-verbal feeling of things, and especially of oneself, whereas consciousness arises with the ability to conceptualise thanks to verbalisation or formal language.[1]

Figure 10.3 defines the different stages of consciousness and awareness. Consciousness takes place on only two levels: representational consciousness (RCS) and self-consciousness (SEC). But there are four ordinary levels of awareness: simple awareness (SIA), unconscious representational awareness (URA), conscious representational awareness (CRA) and self-awareness (SEA).

[1] For a more detailed discussion see Douchamps and Hatayama, 1988.

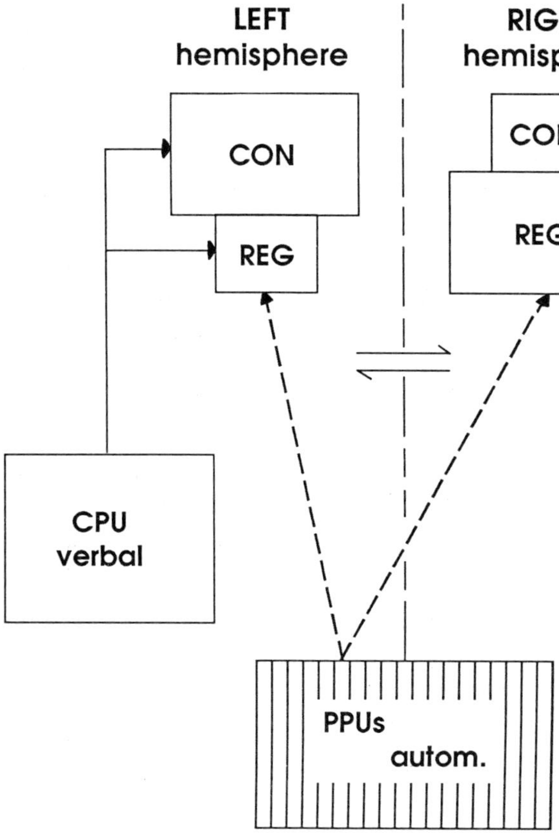


**Figure 10.2 The HOS central structures are duplicated. Each chain contains a central processing unit (CPU), a regulator (REG) and a 'conscioustiser' (CON). Beyond the central processing units, a myriad of small peripheral units (PPUs) generate less complex, automatic behaviours controlled by the regulators of both chains.**

Simple awareness is evoked by simple, stereotyped and automatic processing. Unconscious representational awareness deals with the Freudian and Rankian unconscious. Both representational awareness and representational consciousness are concerned with the perception of the external world. The state of mind concerned with the personal domain is the SEA-SEC state: this is where the Human Operator System becomes involved in the processing programme. Self-awareness arises as an inner sensation of self, while self-consciousness originates from a self-image based on societal rules. A further, completely integrated state occurs when awareness and consciousness are fused (FAW-FCS). This rarely encountered state corresponds to mystical experience.

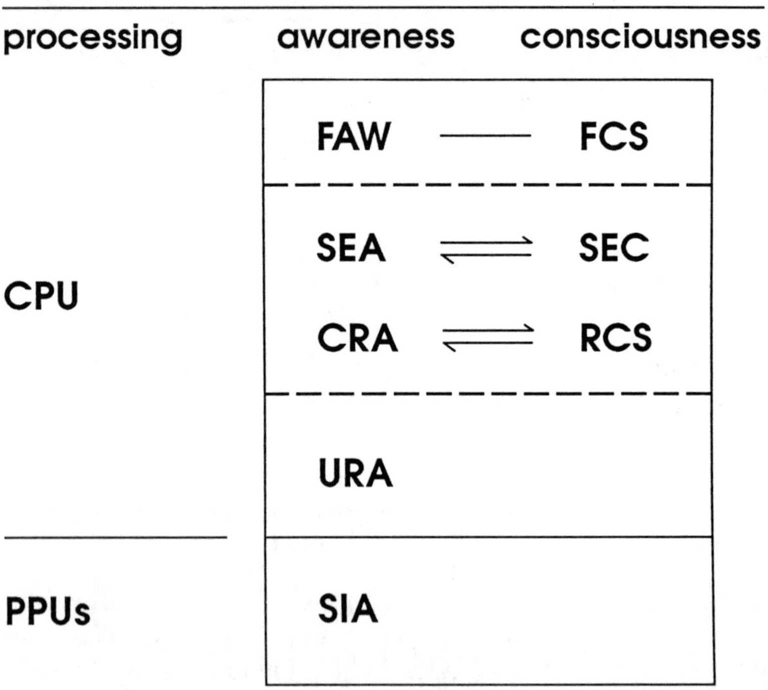


Figure 10.3 Simple awareness (SIA) is linked to automatic functions occurring in the peripheral units of processing (PPUs). More complex processing, taking place in (at least one of) the two central units of processing (CPU), generates unconscious representational awareness (URA, without concomitant consciousness). When the regulator-conscioustiser mechanism is activated, owing to higher HOS systemic powers, such processing gives rise to conscious representational *awareness* (CRA) and representational *consciousness* (RCS). Or, when the personal domain is concerned, such processing gives rise to self-awareness (SEA) and self-consciousness (SEC). Fused awareness and consciousness (FAW-FCS) corresponds to the non-dualistic state of mind found in mystical experience.

## *Stress in our technological civilisation*

Laborit (1986) has emphasised the need for human beings to search for safety through dominance over other members of society. In the light of the way three-dimensional information processing operates, we can envisage three main types of coping behaviour, based primarily on a primitive energetic reaction (ENE), on a more emotional reaction (EMO) or on a more cognitive strategy (LOG).

Each of these types of behaviour has strong and weak points, as summarised in Table 10.1. Essentially, the brain can strengthen its control over its environment in direct proportion to the radius of what we could call a protective bubble which, at best, is composed of three main layers of coping behaviours. However, the bigger the radius of action, the more the control relies on an appropriate use of societal codes.

**Table 10.1. Types of dominance behaviour**

| Main factors | Range of action | Advantage | Drawback |
|---|---|---|---|
| Energy | Individual | Robust | Expensive |
| Emotion | Group | Preventive | Limited |
| Computation | Society | Universal | Dependent |

Source: Douchamps and Hatayama, 1986.

Nowadays professional work and, broadly speaking, social relationships favour cognitive strategies of dominance over emotional or energetic attitudes of coping. The quality, if not the intensity, of the aggression factors has changed, with the coping process evolving in a general intellectualization. Behaviours based on primitive energy or emotion are perceived by individuals as liable to punishment or not effective for ensuring socio-cultural survival. The necessity for commitment in purely logical information exchanges is therefore perceived as unsafe and may elicit ineffective coping behaviours.

## *Reaching for self-recognition*

Self-consciousness – more developed in the dominant, left hemisphere – is the repository of cognitive strategies, and thus can be considered as the indispensable adaptation of the individual brain to societal rules. Self-awareness – more prominent in the non-dominant chain of processing, and hence often minimised and repressed – expresses the intimate (essentially energetical and emotional) needs of the subject, disregarding societal constraints. A solution to the dilemma between individual needs and societal needs can only be found in a better integration of the three-dimensional metrics of the brain achieved by fully balancing the streams of awareness and consciousness. We propose that such an equilibrium emerges through successive, more numerous, and deeper re-structurings of the metacognitive knowledge, a process which we call 'bursts of recognition' (akin to *prises de conscience* in French). But how does this work?

A basic assumption of our HOS model was to consider the human operator system as a dissipative structure (Prigogine, 1980). A characteristic of highly organised dissipative structures is their ability to auto-reorganise, by producing internal fluctuations and a rise in energy. In fact, if a person adopts a viewpoint reflecting the HOS method of thinking – focusing both intuition and rationalisation on the complex, intricate interactions between the self and the world – that individual eventually perceives that all connections are based on circular causalities. At this stage (bursts of recognition), information which was considered as 'noise' when the supervisory system was not operating in this new equilibrium, becomes full of meaning thanks to the new coherence of the system.

## Using the HOS model to benefit society

Turning to practical matters, we can offer two suggestions as to how the HOS model could serve our society.

Firstly, we think the HOS model could serve as a point of reflection on the way we should organise society. In order to respect the balance between our three cerebrotypes, daily life could be centred around three main types of activities, each emphasising an energetic, emotional, or computational approach. The idea is not new. In the Middle Ages, for instance, monks were dividing their daytime activities into thirds, each dedicated to manual work (ENE), intellectual work (LOG), or prayer (EMO). Such a concept could be useful when designing leisure and professional activities in today's society.

Secondly, we note how nowadays many people turn towards Eastern philosopies in the hope of deepening their comprehension of their own minds. The HOS model, founded on scientific principles, highlights the concept of equilibrium proposed by these Eastern systems, but explains it through a descriptive symbolism which is more accessible to Western laymen. Bearing in mind the high stress and anxiety of modern life, if we were to incorporate this heuristic approach to thinking in our educational systems, we may be able to make people aware of both the relativity of most stressors and the richness of life.

# References


Douchamps, J., 'A heuristic model of human performance and its relationship with EEG'. Proceedings of the workshop 'Electroencephalography in Transport Operations', Commission of the European Communities (document IB316-85-03), Cologne, September 1985, pp. 104–117.

Douchamps, J., 'Influence of anxiety on human operational performance: a heuristic approach', Proceedings of the Sixth European Winter Conference on Brain Research, 39, Avoriaz (France), March 1986a.

Douchamps, J., 'A metatheoretic approach of operational performance', in 'Proceedings of the Workshop 'Vigilance: Methods, Models and Regulation', Commission of the European Communities, Dusseldorf (FRG), October 1986b.

Douchamps, J. and Hatayama, T., 'Stress in Technocratic Societies: A Re-Appraisal', *Tohoku Psychologica Folia*, no. 45, 1986, pp. 1–5.

Douchamps, J. and Hatayama, T., 'A Heuristic Model for Human Consciousness', submitted to *Psychologia*.

Laborit, H., *L'Inhibition de l'Action*, Masson, Paris, 1986.

Ledoux, J.E., 'Brain, mind and language', in D.A. Oakley (eds), *Brain and Mind*, London, Methuen, 1985, pp. 197–216.

MacLean, P.D., 'Sensory and perceptive factors in emotional functions of the triune brain', in L. Levi (ed.), *Emotions, their Parameters and Measurement*, Raven Press, New York, 1985, pp. 71–92.

Prigogine, I., *From Being to Becoming*, Freeman, San Francisco, 1980.

Siegrist, J., Siegrist, K. and Weber, I., 'Sociological parameters in studies of breakdown: a selective overview', in Cullen, J. and Siegrist, J. (eds), *Breakdown in Human Adaptation to Stress: towards a Multidisciplinary Approach*, Martinus Nijhoff Publishers, 1984.

Chapter 11

# The whole is greater than the sum of its parts

by Paul Weber

An objective description of the environment relates to material creation, its evolution at different levels and the fundamental laws governing it.

On the other hand, a subjective description of nature from the point of view of the human being includes his relationship with his body and environment, his behaviour, but also his internal environment, i.e. his thoughts, feelings, memories and consciousness as such.

In order to cope with the environmental crisis today, it is necessary to re-integrate the objective and subjective approaches to nature.

## Environment

Environment is what we call that which surrounds us. Our five senses enable us to perceive both human society, with its myriad industrial and cultural goods, and the natural environment, consisting of galaxies, stars, planets, stones, plants, animals and so forth. As children, we tend to experience our surroundings in a magical, intuitive fashion; later on, as our minds develop, this often gives way to a more mechanical, rational world view.

Alternatively, we may describe the objective environment in more abstract terms. We can sharpen our senses by using technology, for example, telescopes or microscopes. Experimentally validated scientific theory widens our horizons when it comes to understanding nature. In this century alone, what was a mechanistic and linear world view has taken a probabilistic, non-linear turn under the successive development of the general theory of relativity, quantum mechanics, quantum-chrono-dynamics and the complex theory of relativity. Jean E. Charon (1987) has literally put us in the picture. The different theories are simply different steps in the process of describing nature objectively. They are ways of looking at the same objects at different stages.

From time immemorial, scientists have felt the need to integrate different theories. Newton was the first to produce such a synthesis, describing the movement of a body on earth and that of celestial objects in a single, simple equation. Maxwell then succeeded in expressing the phenomena of electricity and magnetism in a single theory. Subsequently, field theories were used to combine weak force and electromagnetic force. Now it seems that the final hurdles standing in the path of a single 'unified field theory' are being overcome.

Just as nature can be described in a series of steps, complementary ways of viewing reality are also beginning to emerge, as depicted in Figure 11.1. Each individual part or building block of nature would seem to contain

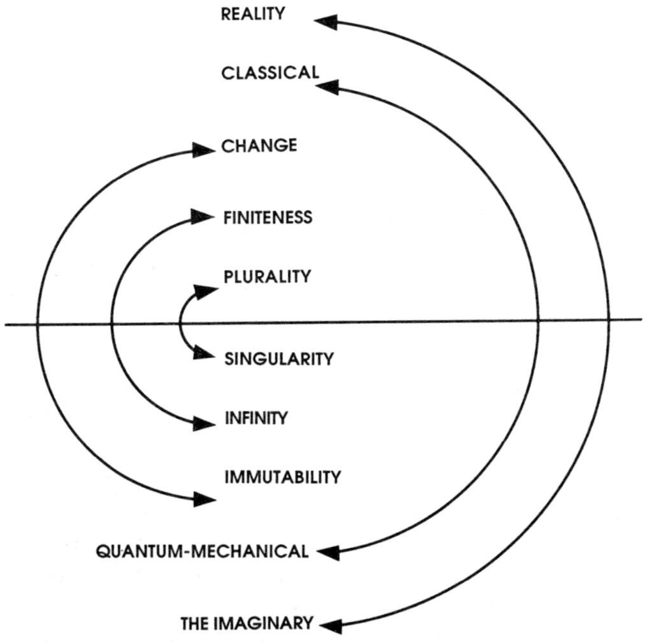


**Figure 11.1 Complementary ways of viewing reality**

within it the full potential of the whole. What we perceive as the plurality of creation is in fact nothing but the manifestation of various aspects of the unified field. We can best visualize this by taking a look at the development of the cosmos according to the Big Bang theory, (Fritsch, 1983), as illustrated in Figure 11.2.

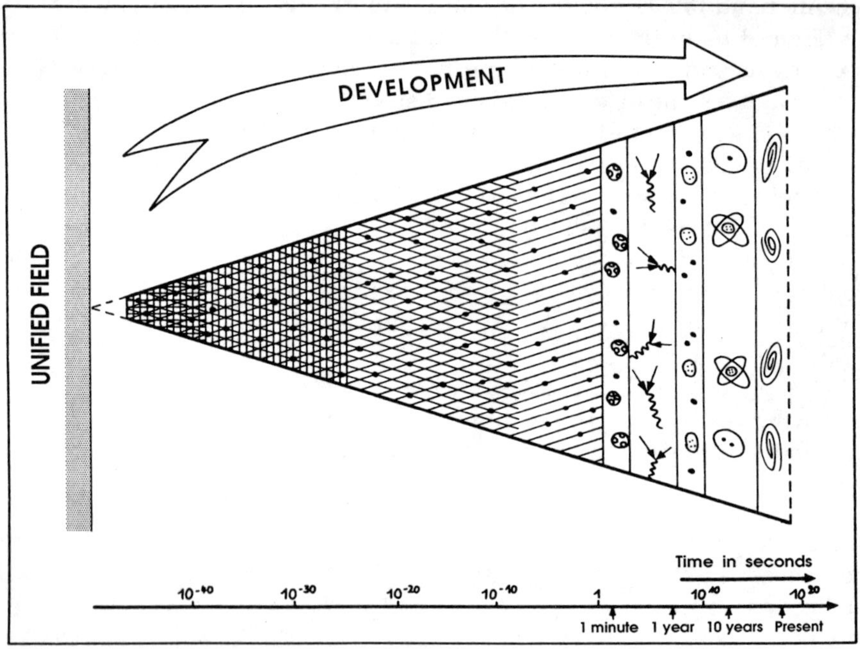


**Figure 11.2 Development of the cosmos**

Space and time condense from the unified field after the Big Bang. As the spontaneous and sequential breaking of this perfect symmetry gathers momentum, first there emerge the four energy fields and the elementary particles, then atoms and molecules, bio-macro-molecules, cells, tissues and organs, organic systems and finally human beings. All this takes some fifteen billion years to complete. Microcosm and macrocosm obey the same fundamental law of nature. Each part contains the whole. Opposites exist in equilibrium or else complete each other.

Nature is bent on achieving ever higher and increasingly complex forms of organisation and, subjectively speaking, strives towards esthetic and functional perfection. Nature, in other words, wants to unfold her full potential. Human activity can be detrimental to steady-state equilibrium in nature. The effects of human interference at the various levels depend on how well people understand nature's ways in objective terms, as we can see below.

| Nature at various levels | Human activity |
|---|---|
| • Animals | • Stock-farming, hunting and fishing, genetic engineering |
| • Plants | • Forestry and farming |
| • Bio-macro-molecules | • Biotechnology, biogenetics |
| • Atoms and molecules | • Ozone, $CO_2$, chemical production |
| • Elementary particles | • Nuclear fission, nuclear fusion |
| • Energy fields | • Laser, radio, television, radar, gravity converter |

Human activity only really becomes an environmental hazard when it is based on imperfect knowledge and understanding, as it then upsets the natural steady-state equilibrium. Interrupted cycles result in solid waste, waste water, polluted air, waste heat – a whole litany of environmental complaints, an accumulation of nuisances, simply because nature's own degradation and recycling mechanisms cannot keep pace or fail altogether. Feedback and synergism further intensify the consequences, so that by now the havoc wrought by human clumsiness on Earth's atmosphere, its oceans and its land masses defies computation.

## Human beings

Humans perceive the environment through the five senses. They interpret their sensory impressions by using their brains, so brain physiology and intellect come into play. Albert Einstein once said that human beings use only five to ten per cent of their brain potential. The remaining ninety per cent make up what psychologists call the subconscious, the unconscious or the soul. Intellect and reasoning power play a connecting and integrating role. A symbol may help to bring this idea into focus. Look at the mobile in Figure 11.3.

The mobile is attached to the ceiling by a thread, and it revolves in time and space. Individual units of creation – such as star systems, trees, aquatic systems, human beings or the products of civilisation – exist in equilibrium. When human action shatters that equilibrium, the weights shift and the environment has to adjust to regain its balance. If, for example, the earth's forests were to disappear, nature would have to take drastic remedial action or the entire mobile would get hopelessly entangled in its own threads.

Possibly the greatest single man-made cause of disequilibrium in nature's mobile is that people's environmental awareness leaves much to be desired. We have not yet learned to recognise nature's many features and have only a feeble grasp of the way in which they interact. Generally people are only dimly aware of being an integral part of the cosmic mobile themselves.

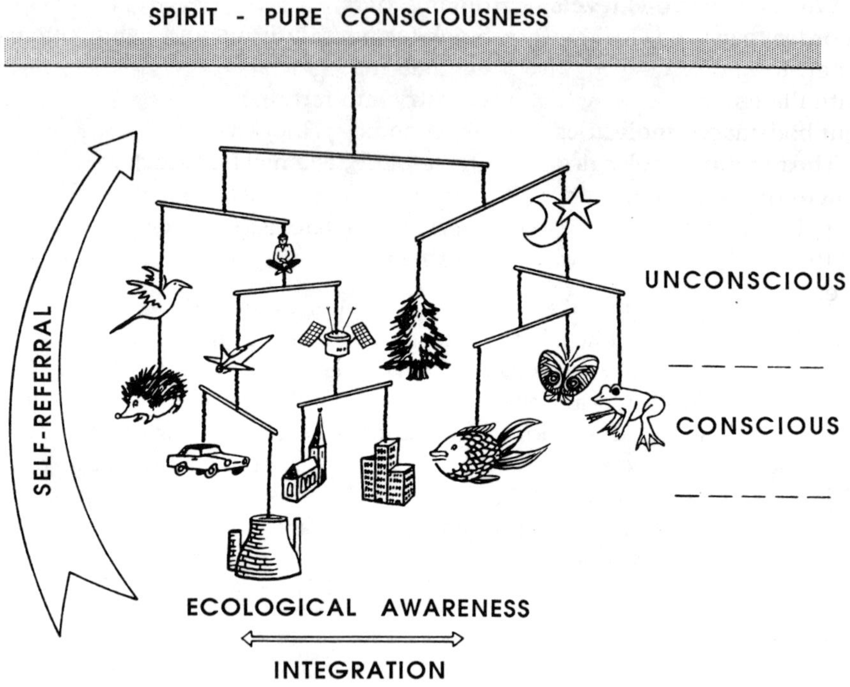


**Figure 11.3 Subjectivity: spiritual progress**

'Here am "I"', we say, 'and there is the "environment"'. This dichotomy is the rule by which we live. There are few who will say: '"I" am part of the whole, and that is my "con-vironment": the world of which I am part and which co-exists on equal terms.' The ecologically aware reject the egotistical 'I' barricaded inside their own skin and view people as irrevocably part and parcel of nature.

Since the human mind boggles at the staggering diversity of nature and cannot grasp its myriad cross-relationships, we feel the need to simplify things by imposing a more abstract structure. Nothing could be more natural. So just as, when examining nature, we found we could formulate fundamentals in abstract terms by means of quantum mechanics, when considering the conditions of human life the great philosophers and spiritual teachers of all cultures and all times (for example, Shankara, Plato, Patanjali, Meister Eckhart, Spinoza and Schelling) have commended withdrawal from the sensory impressions and a sort of effortless, non-intellectual introspection in order to achieve self-awareness. This knowledge of the transcendental ego was for them the prerequisite for gaining stability, confidence and fulfilment in life.

We need such self-referral through methods like deep meditation or yoga in order to get the world into perspective, to understand ourselves and each other, to know the 'self' and make sense of and improve our relationship with the environment, which we may define in this context as the 'non-self' (our body and surroundings).

Those who attempt the subjective voyage of self-discovery, where all hinges on personal experience, should find themselves proceeding, step by step, to loftier and increasingly abstract strata of awareness. Wise men tell us that everybody can gradually achieve awareness of the unconscious and even, perhaps, experience the Greek ideal of unity or oneness of body, mind and soul. In terms of our mobile, this would mean 'seeing' the ceiling, the threads and the objects hanging by them as a single whole – as one-and-the-same thing.

The world's spiritual leaders and philosophers have always argued that imperfect self-referral or imperfect communion with the inner self produces stress in the 'threads of the mobile'. It leads to unnatural or erroneous behaviour, which in turn creates problems for the individual or for the community as a whole, as shown in Figure 11.4.

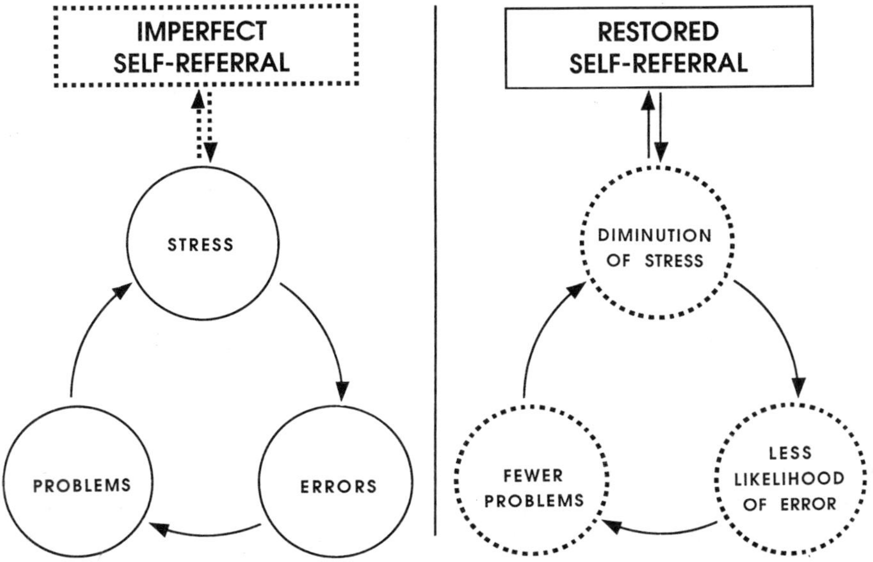


**Figure 11.4 Imperfect and restored self-referral**

A handful of scientists have introduced us to the world of quantum and relativity; high technology has given us the corresponding instruments of power. This means that an ever greater number of environmentally unaware people can, wittingly or unwittingly, abuse that power. To act without surveying the consequences of action is irresponsible, unethical, immoral and a recipe for disaster. We must make sure that subjective self-knowledge keeps pace with objective science. The tenets of wise men of the past and the quantum philosophy of latter-day scientists must be integrated; our spiritual potential must be given more scope. Then we can decide in which way and at which level we need to learn more about behaving in a manner that will create a compatible relationship between people and environment.

## Health

Health is a factor which helps to determine the relationship between the human being and his environment. It is interesting to look at the cycle of matter between the two. To stay alive for twenty-four hours, a human being needs some eight kilos of air, two kilos of liquid and one kilo of solid food. The most important ingredient is clean air, unfouled by cigarette smoke and atmospheric pollution.

The interaction of oxygen and carbon dioxide between human and plant life amply illustrates our mutual dependence: what is waste to one is nourishment to the other. This natural equilibrium is achieved so rapidly that human atoms become environment and environment becomes a human body in the space of a single year. In other words, the body we inhabit today did not exist a year ago. Ninety-eight per cent of its atoms were still elsewhere in the environment.

Some experts maintain that:

- the skeleton changes once every three months,
- the skin once a month,
- the liver once every six weeks,
- the mucous lining of the stomach once every eight days, and
- the brain cells once a year.

Medicine shows us how the different organs of the body interact; ecology does the same for the 'organs' of nature. Our intellect has found two complementary ways of husbanding health. On the one hand there is allopathy or scientific healing, which wields an array of increasingly sophisticated instruments to cope with the symptoms of disease in our bodies. On the other hand we have natural healing, which seeks to achieve an 'original' balance between all parts of the organism and a free flow of energy within the whole.

Medicine's counterparts in terms of environmental protection would be, respectively, objective scientific definition and subjective empirical recognition of the laws of nature. Fever, smoker's lung, the accumulation of residues in the body, circulatory problems caused by thickening of the arteries, blunting of the faculties, cancer growths and acquired immune deficiency syndrome (AIDS) are to medicine what the greenhouse effect on climate, depletion of the ozone layer, air pollution, poisoned waste, water pollution, man-made 'correction' of rivers, the extinction of species, overpopulation and the decline of nature's regenerative powers are to environmental protection.

There is an Indian proverb which says: 'A well-fed person needs no medicine; an ill-nourished one needs none either'. Applied to the environment, this might read: 'A person who respects the laws of nature needs no environmental protection; a person who spurns nature will not be saved by environmental protection.'

The proverb pays homage to old Ayurvedic wisdom, which holds that a malady should be extirpated at source for it to be vanquished forever. Symptomatic treatment is part-healing with side effects. Treating forest soil with lime to revive moribund trees while allowing air pollution to go unchecked is like treating acid stomach with sodium bicarbonate without prescribing a change of diet.

I would define the pursuit of health in human beings and in nature as seeking a state of equilibrium between all parts. This would dovetail with the definition adopted by the World Health Organization in its constitution in 1946: Health is a state of complete physical, mental and social well-being, not merely the absence of disease or disability.

By that definition, we are currently violating the laws of nature in three major areas: (1) We interrupted the cycle of matter in its three phases: growth, utilisation and degradation (or birth, life and death). (2) We have forgotten that by the law of least action, ecology and economy are complementary – not contradictory – values. (3) Too few of us have learned that objective development and subjective self-referral can coalesce to form a new whole.

So when speaking of people living compatibly in good health within the environment, polarity is not at issue. We are not talking about 'either/or' but about 'as well as': evolution *and* self-referral, reductionism *and* holism, object *and* subject, having *and* being, the treatment of symptoms *and* causes, fire-fighting *and* emergency planning, freedom of the individual *and* regard for fellow human beings, expansion *and* reintegration, human health *and* the health of the 'con-vironment' ... .

## Coping with crisis

The problems we encounter in the environment and in failing human health are merely the symptoms of a deeper crisis. They are part of a global crisis

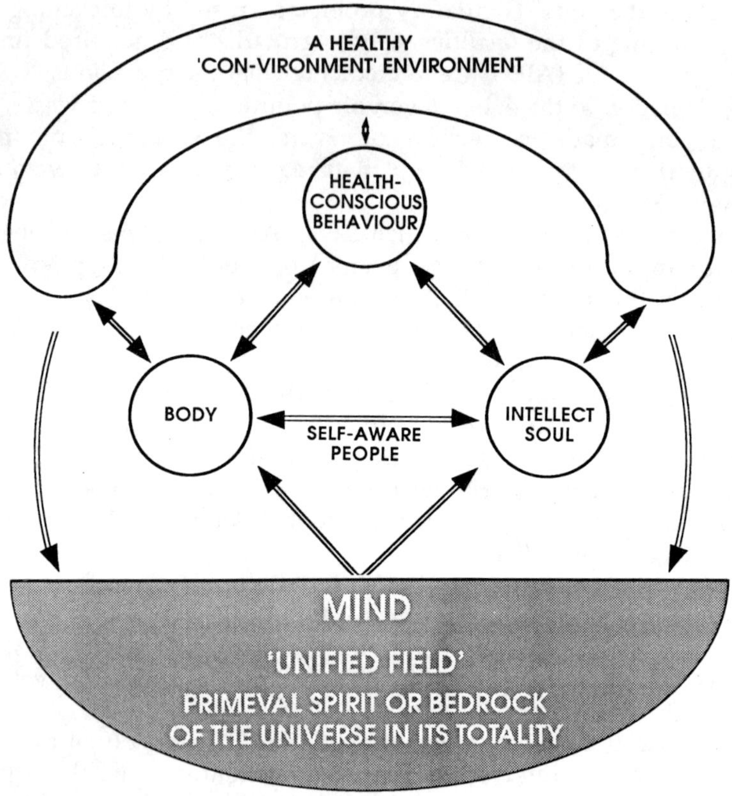


**Figure 11.5 The whole is greater than the sum of its parts**

involving the environment, health, the economy, finance, the third world, armaments, genetic engineering, nuclear technology, etc.

It is the power – or rather the power*lessness* – of human consciousness itself which must ultimately be brought to book for precipitating our crisis. Our consciousness shies away from admitting that it, and only it, darkens our perceptions and misleads our behaviour. Indeed, how could it do otherwise, scarcely knowing itself.

We surmise that we are fairly ignorant about ourselves and seek to compensate through our actions in the objective world. The result has been soaring energy consumption and unprecedented pillaging of other raw materials, through which we effect lasting and wholly uncalled for change in the world.

We can only hope to come to grips with the crisis if we revert to the subjective. Our economic goods, our cultural goods, the world we have 'made' are merely the objective mirror of our partial awareness of ourselves.

Unless human beings will establish harmony and peace in their inner selves through the process of self-referral and regular exposure to the silence which lies deep inside of them, no objective approach alone can solve the problems of health and environment which we face today.

The fragmented thinking of the human has led to decisions and activities which have disrupted the balance in nature. We have created an unhealthy whole by weakening so many of its parts (air, water, earth, plants, animals and ourselves). Holistic thinking and feeling is necessary in order to re-establish a healthy whole which is greater than the sum of its parts.

## References

Charon, Jean E., *Der Sündenfall der Evolution*, Paul Zsolnay, 1987.

Fritsch, Harold, *Bild der Wissenschaft*, no. 6, 1983.

# Part II

# Scientists and Civilisation Diseases

Chapter 12

# Civilisation diseases, time and space

by Francisco Chavarria

It would be impossible to list all civilisation diseases here, but what follows is a selection, and includes those groups which are the highest causes of mortality in the Western world:

- cardio-vascular diseases (heart attacks, high blood pressure)
- cancer
- accidents (work and traffic)
- job-related illnesses
- toxicopathology (pesticides, food additives, preservatives, colourants etc.)
- psychological and behaviour disorders (depression, aggressiveness, anxiety, etc.)
- immune-deficiency illnesses (AIDS)
- allergies
- genetic disorders (chromosome damage)
- social disorders (terrorism etc.).

In Spain, where I work, the mortality rate per 100,000 inhabitants from cardio-vascular disease is fifty, from cancer twenty and from accidents seven. Below I shall look at each of these in turn.

## *Cardio-vascular disease*

This is the primary cause of mortality in the developed world. In Spain it accounts for fifty per cent of all deaths.[1] Twenty per cent of the population is affected by high blood pressure and there are:

- 6,000 cases of congenital heart disease per year
- 20, 000 new cases of coronary thrombosis per year
- 160 new cases of strokes per 100,000 inhabitants per year
- one death through heart attacks every thirty minutes.

These figures give us some idea of the problem and force us to face the risk factors involved – tobacco, eating habits, obesity, pollution, stress, etc. – which when combined give a typical overview of our civilisation.

## *Cancer*

For cancer, civilisational factors shaping the natural and cultural environment are second only to genetic factors. There are general, natural risk factors such as food, hormones, certain products of the intermediary metabolism, solar radiation, etc., and artificial ones such as job-related risks, technology, pollution, medicines, chemicals, agriculture, industry, sport, creature comforts, cultural habits (tobacco, alcohol) and certain leisure atmospheres (discotheques, pubs, etc.).[2] Tobacco alone is the most important factor in bronchopulmonary cancer, both in active and passive smokers. Tobacco smoke contains at least twelve chemical carcinogenic substances. Alcohol is not carcinogenic but is an additional risk, especially when associated with tobacco. Together they increase significantly the number of cancers of the larynx, mouth, liver, bladder, oesophagus and stomach.

Exogenous agents account for eighty to ninety per cent of all etiological factors and fifty to eighty per cent of these are chemicals and physical agents.

In Spain cancer accounts for about twenty per cent of all deaths.[3] But types of cancer are distributed differently among men and women, as shown in Table 12.1. It is clear that cancer is a major civilisation disease, but progress is being made. The average total cure rate for cancer is now forty-five to fifty per cent.

---

1 'Incidentia se las enfermedades cardiovasculares en España, *F. Hispana de Cardiologia*, 1986.

2 Ministerio de Sanidad y Consumo, *Libro Blanco para la Planificacion Global de la Oncología en España*, (forthcoming).

3 Ibid.

Table 12.1 Types of cancer in men and women in Spain

| Men | | Women | |
|---|---|---|---|
| Lungs | 14.0 % | Breast | 33.4 % |
| Skin | 12.6 % | Skin | 11.4 % |
| Larynx | 12.3 % | Uterus | 9.4 % |
| Blabber | 8.1 % | Cervix | 5.7 % |
| Stomach | 6.9 % | Stomach | 4.4 % |
| Prostate | 3.8 % | Rectum | 4.1 % |
| Rectum | 3.5 % | Ovaries | 2.8 % |
| Oesophagus | 3.1 % | Haemopoiesitic S. | 2.5 % |
| Colon | 2.7 % | Colon | 2.2 % |
| Hematopoietic and Lymphatic systems | 2.2 % | Lungs | 1.9 % |

Source: Figures for 1981: Fundación Científica de la A.E.C.C., 'Datos estadisticos y epidemiológicos del Cáncer en España; Situación Actual', *Informa XIV*, 1987.

## *Job-related illnesses and accidents*

In 1982 the following job-related illnesses were recorded in Spain.[4]

| | |
|---|---|
| by physical agents | 3,756 |
| by chemical agents (notably derivatives of benzene, anilines, nitrosamines, pesticides, vinyl chloride, carbon sulphide, phosphorus etc.) | 360 |
| by biological agents | 225 |

Among the physical agents, noise (2,013) and repetitive movements (1,358) were the highest cause of illness, but other factors are also important: ultraviolet radiation, abnormal mechanical pressure, vibrations, radiant energy, microwaves, etc.

According to the Spanish Ministry of Work and Social Security the total number of accidents in the workplace dropped between 1977 and 1986, but it is interesting to note that in Madrid between September 1986 and September 1987 there was a 19.08 per cent increase in the number of minor

4 Sanchez Ramos, E. and Sanchez Gomez, E., 'Enfermedades profesionales en España', *Salud y Trabajo*, vol. 50, nos. 38–43, 1985, nos. 15–22, 1986.

accidents and a 60 per cent increase in the number of accidental deaths.
Accidents also increased differently according to profession:

| | |
|---|---|
| Agriculture: | 26.92 per cent |
| Industry: | 20.97 per cent |
| Construction: | 30.05 per cent |
| Services: | 15.35 per cent. |

### *Road accidents*

Road accidents are a major cause of death in the developed world. In Spain there was a twenty per cent increase in the total number of accidents between 1985 and 1986, and an eight per cent increase in the total number of victims.[5] The figures in Table 12.2 are for 1986 in Spain.

**Table 12.2 Victims of road accidents in Spain, 1986**

| | |
|---|---|
| **Total number of accidents with victims** | |
| In towns | 45,766 |
| Out of towns | 41,937 |
| **Total number of victims** | |
| Injured | 137,145 |
| Killed | 5,419 |
| in towns | 988 |
| out of towns | 4,431 |

## The framework of civilisation diseases

I have looked briefly at three types of civilisation disease to illustrate their particularities and the problems posed to our societies by them. But we must study civilisation diseases not only in order to know and treat them better, but also to discover their reason for being. We need to study the framework in which they fit and discover the meaning of all the elements in play and the possible correlations between them.

Perhaps then we should see civilisation diseases not as diseases at all but symptoms of the disease of civilisation itself. To do this we have to ask

5 Direccíon General de Tráfico, Datos Estadísticos referentes a 1985 y 1986; López Alonso, E.J., 'Conducir es convivir', *La Caja*, no. 73, 1987, pp. 16–18.

ourselves what we mean by 'civilisation'. For me, it is the effective consequence of human nature. But each civilisation, in its time and space, is a crossroads of biology, ecology and culture, and it is not possible to look at certain of its components without taking the whole into account.

Life and environment are part of time and space and their possible disorders can be expressed as civilisation diseases. Nearly all the risk factors I discussed earlier, both natural and artificial, have cultural – and therefore civilisational – connotations. They all act through accumulation in biological space and time and in synchronisation with cosmic space and time – which themselves act to condition and modulate the total real risk. For most cancers, for instance, we can certainly talk about multifactorial risk. To try to understand accumulation and the concept of unity between life and environment, however, we need to look briefly at three concepts: functional synchronisation, time and space.

## *Functional synchronisation, time and space*

Biological structures and the environment are organised into structural bioecology, in which the edges of each component relate rather than separate. Even if there is separation, there is no real compartmentalization because each structure is linked to those below and above to make systematic integration possible. But in biology, no organic integration is possible outside of what we might call *functional synchronisation.*

If organic integration occurs in three-dimensional space, then functional synchronisation involves a fourth dimension: time. Organisation, integration and synchronisation become the most important factors needed to reach the complete system. Life in general, and human life in particular, can therefore be seen as open dynamic systems structured according to relative organic spaces with functional particularities, and evolving both in biological time and cosmic space and time.

From a strictly biological point of view, there are three forms of time: organic, cosmic and real time. Organic time is neuronal, cellular, hormonal, metabolic, etc. and cosmic time is night, day, weeks, months, seasons and years. Organic time always straddles cosmic time. Real time is a synchronisation of organic and cosmic time. In this way life moves in real time through birth, youth, age, maturity, reproduction, ageing and death. When the concept of time is added to biology, we have *chronobiology.*

There are four forms of space: organic, cosmic, structural and real. Traditionally the body and its external environment together make up organic space and are integrated into the 'environment' – in the widest sense of the word – in cosmic space. But in modern anthropology, there is also structural space, where nature and culture integrate So real space can be seen as the synchronisation of organic, cosmic and structural space.

There can never be empty space, therefore, but instead the synchronised platform of real space where multiple and varied interaction takes place.

By integrating time and space into biology we can envisage a four-dimensional organisation where reality determines the structure of space. The environment becomes an integrated system where the space between things is no less real than the things themselves in the dynamics which time imposes. In the last analysis, energy would link the micro- and the macrocosm. Biology would become *cosmobiology*, with reality a vectorial solution between need and probability in each given time and space.

In this light, civilisation diseases can be seen as the expression of an eco-anthropo-pathology resulting from the relationship between man and environment in time and space, and where synchronisation would be the equivalent of a sort of universal cosmic solidarity.

Chapter 13

# Nutrition and health: there is a future

by Joseph Hautvast

From the point of view of nutrition, Europe is a fascinating region, with large differences in dietary and culinary practices. There are differences in the contributions of fat and carbohydrates in the diet; different kinds of fats and oils are eaten; people eat different kinds and amounts of vegetables; and there are the well-known differences in the use of alcoholic beverages and liquors.

More than a century ago specialists in Europe were already trying to relate the nutritional quality of national diets with national performance and progress. In the first part of this century it gradually became clear that food constituents – such as energy, vitamins and trace elements – play a very important role in the maintenance of health and in the prevention of diseases. Although scientific progress in this field was very impressive, application of the knowledge was still far from ideal due to poor living conditions, and economic and environmental stresses. In the decades before 1940, the working class was often consuming nutritionally poor diets which could cause deficiency diseases or a reduced resistance to infectious diseases. For many groups of Europeans, the Second World War was a nutritional disaster; we recall, for example, the documented evidence of the death by starvation of the Jewish people in the Warsaw ghetto and the Dutch Famine in the winter of 1944–45.

After the war a unique situation gradually developed: for the first time in European history, despite the large population, more than enough food became available for almost everybody. In addition, a fantastic and unbelievable diversity of processed foods appeared in markets and in shops. For those who remember the period before the Second World War, it must seem strange that even the present diversity and abundance of food is causing considerable health problems. Thus we need to discuss and explain the question of good nutrition, analyse dietary practices in relation to health, and provide dietary recommendations which will give maximum support for human health.

## Nutrition and health in Europe

Since 1950, evidence began to mount that intake levels of different nutrients might be linked to certain health risks and diseases – like cardio-vascular diseases, gallstones, obesity, hypertension, diabetes and cancers of the lung, stomach and large intestines. These diseases are not only a great burden on health services and on human and financial resources in Europe, but are also often a cause of unexpected family tragedy and disruption due to premature mortality. Two of the most prevalent diseases causing high mortality within Europe are cardio-vascular diseases and cancer. A review of the role of nutrition in these diseases leads to the conclusion that changes in dietary patterns are truly indicated.

### *Nutrition and cardio-vascular diseases*

Within Europe we observe considerable differences and even a north-south gradient in the standardised mortality rate by ischemic heart diseases (due to obstruction of the inflow of arterial blood). The three main causes of cardio-vascular diseases are smoking, high blood pressure and high blood cholesterol levels. But there is also some evidence that nutritional factors – like sodium, magnesium, calcium and obesity – play a role in balancing the level of blood pressure. The level of blood cholesterol, on the other hand, can be influenced by changes in the diet, especially in the amounts and kinds of fat eaten.

It is therefore not very surprising that the WHO Expert Committee on Prevention of Coronary Heart Disease in 1986 decided that nutrition should be the principal area for action. Seeing a need to reduce the average blood cholesterol level in many populations and to prevent future rises in others, the Committee recommended a reduction of saturated fat intake to about 30 per cent of total fat intake and to no more than about 10 per cent of an individual's total energy intake. In addition, it recommended reduced intake of salt, dietary cholesterol, and alcohol.

Over the past ten to fifteen years, many non-governmental organisations, like heart foundations, had already given such dietary recommendations; and in recent years governments have also been getting involved in this issue. The difference is that now this involvement is *action-oriented* rather than only education-oriented. Such approaches are justified, as mounting evidence from experimental research and from community projects supports the view that the major cardio-vascular diseases are substantially preventable. That changes in mortality rates due to cardio-vascular diseases *do* take place is shown in Table 13.1.

**Table 13.1 Percentage change over a ten-year period in age-standardised mortality rates from cardio-vascular diseases in adults aged 40–69 years**

| Country | Period | Cardio-vascular diseases | |
|---|---|---|---|
| | | *male* | *female* |
| France | 1971–81 | -23 | -35 |
| Finland | 1970–80 | -20 | -40 |
| England, Wales | 1972–82 | -17 | -20 |
| Netherlands | 1972–82 | -16 | -23 |
| Norway | 1972–82 | -10 | -25 |
| Italy | 1970–80 | -9 | -28 |
| Yugoslavia | 1971–81 | +24 | +13 |
| Hungary | 1972–82 | +33 | +3 |

Source: WHO Technical Report Series 732, 1986.

The decline of mortality can, of course, not be ascribed only to better nutrition: the advances in medical technologies and the reduction in smoking are of comparable importance. Yet the increase in cardio-vascular mortality in countries like Hungary and Yugoslavia is very likely due to the fact that the recommended dietary changes, especially with regard to the fat component, have not yet taken place in these countries. We can be very sure that such a decline can be expected in these countries as soon as dietary changes are introduced. Thus we might conclude that the epidemics of cardio-vascular diseases in the second half of the twentieth century will wane in the future.

## *Nutrition and cancer*

The fight against cancer is becoming the big health issue of the coming decades. Cancer is the second main cause of death in industrialised countries. But sadly the wealth of our knowledge about the causes and prevention of cardio-vascular diseases is equal to the limitation of our scientific information about the causes and prevention of cancer. The main scientific questions at present are to what extent cancers are avoidable and, if so, how to avoid them? At present we are really at an interface between information based on evidence from epidemiological studies and the unknown results of clinical trials now in progress whose conclusions will not become available until the 1990s or later.

The classic document on avoidability of cancer was written by Richard Doll and Richard Peto in 1981. According to them much evidence already exists on the avoidability of cancer. They summarised information under the following four headings:

1. *There are clear differences in cancer incidences between communities.* For example, Japanese have much higher incidence rates for stomach cancer than Europeans; Seventh-Day Adventists experience low incidence rates for cancers of the gastrointestinal system.

2. *Migrants show different incidences of cancer compared to the same ethnic groups who do not migrate.* The famous example is the Japanese migrants to Hawaii. Instead of being like the Japanese living in Japan, most cancer rates for the migrants are becoming like those of the Caucasian residents in Hawaii.

3. *Cancer incidences are changing over time.* The sharp decline of stomach cancer in the past decades and the strong increase of breast cancer are well-known examples.

4. *Information is available about exposure of people to chemical substances or their use in animal experiments.* This leads to more information regarding the identification of the causes of cancer.

Doll and Peto made estimates of various risks of cancer that can be attributable to different classes of environmental agents (Table 13.2.).

The estimates presented in the table underline the need to pay more attention to dietary factors in any search for the cause of cancer. But it is difficult to formulate as firm a conclusion based upon nutrition as we have done when discussing prevention of cardio-vascular diseases. The basic question now is whether we can consider that the available indirect and circumstantial evidence linking diet and cancer is of sufficiently high quality to formulate provisional dietary recommendations, or whether this approach is unethical because recommendations should be based upon unequivocally proved findings. The World Health Organization, the European Community and many national governments have chosen the first option. They have formulated interim dietary guidelines which are not likely to have harmful effects and which have a good possibility of reducing the risk of the major cancers induced by diet.

For example, in 1987 the European Community launched a programme called *Europe Against Cancer,* covering cancer prevention, health education, public information and other fields. The programme's action plan is composed of what is termed ten simple rules, four of which are concerned with nutrition:

- moderate consumption of alcoholic drinks
- eat sufficient fresh fruits and vegetables
- eat sufficient cereals with a high fibre content
- eat low fat foods and avoid becoming overweight.

Other rules relate to smoking, exposure to the sun, and early detection of certain cancers. The application of these interim dietary guidelines and the research and clinical trials on aetiology, prevention and cure of cancers hold the promise that the fight against cancer will become a successful programme in the next century.

**Table 13.2 Risks of cancer attributable to various environmental agents**

| Factor or class of factors | Per cent of all cancer deaths | |
|---|---|---|
| | Best estimate | Range of acceptable estimates |
| Diet | 35 | 10–70 |
| Tobacco | 30 | 25–40 |
| Infection | 10? | 1 – ? |
| Reproduction, sexuality | 7 | 1 –13 |
| Occupation | 4 | 2 – 8 |
| Alcohol | 3 | 2 – 4 |
| Geophysical factors | 3 | 2 – 4 |
| Pollution | 2 | <1 – 5 |
| Medicines/medical treatments | 1 | 0.5 – 3 |
| Food additives | <1 | -5 – 2 |
| Industrial products | <1 | <1 – 2 |
| Unknown | ? | ? |

## The role of nutrition in maintaining good health

Cavities, obesity, gallstones, allergies, rheumatoid arthrosis, and perhaps migraine headaches are also diseases in which nutrition plays a more or less prominent role. Another area which also needs great attention is the nutritional care of the elderly. In the next decade the elderly population in the western world will be about 12–14 per cent of the total. These unique developments regarding increased life expectancy urgently call for nutritional guidelines to maintain good health and unimpaired mental and physical performances as long as possible. That nutrition plays an important role in this age group can hardly be denied; whether the dietary recommendations should be more specific is not yet known. Ongoing research will perhaps provide some of the answers in the next decade. But from a nutritional health perspective we are already sure that in this age group too, adequate nutrition will add life to years and not only years to life.

Thus there is broad evidence that nutrition is an important determinant of health, and in many countries 'Guidelines for a Healthy Diet' have been formulated. The messages of these dietary guidelines can be summarised as follows:

- eat a variety of foods
- maintain an adequate body weight
- reduce fat intake, especially of saturated fat
- increase carbohydrate intake
- decrease sugar, cholesterol and salt intake
- increase dietary fibre intake
- avoid excessive alcohol intake.

These suggested dietary changes do not look new or impressive. Still, we foresee a gradual breakthrough in public opinion and attitudes towards their application. Moreover, we believe that in the coming decade there will be impressive achievements in the field of nutritional health. Our belief is based on a number of observations:

- the available and still growing scientific evidence that dietary changes do indeed support good health;
- growing political agreement, especially in agricultural policies, on the importance of the nutritional quality of a diet, irrespective of a country's domestic products;
- growing involvement and enthusiasm of the food processing industry in bringing fast foods with less fat and more carbohydrates onto the market;
- the growing interest of the medical profession in using diet as a therapy along with medicines;
- frequent and continuing media attention to food and nutrition issues (although too often featuring food faddism instead of health nutrition!);
- the growing awareness and interest of consumers in discussing food and composing diets which follow the recommended guidelines.

The recommended dietary changes do not mean a change to a completely different diet. Often they only involve a slight adaptation of the diet presently eaten. For example, in my country, the Netherlands, the guidelines mean that we should stop eating 100 grams of fat a day and change to 80–85 grams. Such a small restriction in fat intake should be compensated by eating somewhat more carbohydrates.

Such targets of dietary change will probably be reached in the coming decade. Consequently, other nutritional targets may also be introduced successfully. Therefore the statement 'nutrition and health: there is a future' is not a palatable dream, but a strong reality.

## Reference

*The Causes of Cancer*, Oxford Medical Publications, Oxford University Press, 1981.

Chapter 14

# The biology of cerebral ageing

by Corneliu Giurgea

Howard Fast, the American writer, has this image in one of his latest novels: 'Old age is a country you never visit until you come to settle there.' But we must not forget that every country has lots of different places in it and it is a good idea to choose the one that suits you the most, the one that enables you to exploit your resources to the full. This is particularly true of cerebral ageing, and it is not surprising that it is high on the World Health Organization's list of priorities, not only because of its medical, but also of its socio-economic, psychological, deontological and moral aspects.

In ancient Rome life expectancy at birth was twenty. In the United States today, for men and women combined, it is seventy-nine. In 1950, the number of years a sixty-five year old man could expect to live was twelve and a woman of the same age, thirteen. In 1980, it was fifteen years for men and twenty for women. In 1984 the over-eighties numbered 5.6 million. In the year 2000, there will be more than ten million. By the same year, worldwide, there will be twenty-four million more over-eighties than now (Domino et al., 1978). The women:men ratio of the same age group in 2000 will be 2:1, as will the elderly:teenager ratio. Such an evolution in life expectancy will be accompanied by changes in our perception of old age itself, and the place of the elderly in our societies. The implications are wide-ranging. There will perhaps be fewer adverts for jeans and hamburgers and more for rest homes and universities for the elderly. We are also going to witness an increase in the number of patients with *senile dementia* and a variety of physical handicaps, and this is going to put a bigger and bigger burden on society in general and families in particular.

There is a growing acceptance amongst most specialists that pathological cerebral ageing is not the inexorable fate of the physiological ageing of the brain. That in fact there is more of a break than a continuity between the two. However, we do not yet know the real causes – the physiopathological mechanism – of physiological cerebral ageing, any more than we know those for ageing in general. We are reminded of the French professor of medicine, Bichat's, difficulty when asked to define life: 'That whole set of processes which opposes death'.

## What is ageing?

Ageing is a relatively slow process which follows a genetic programme written by the species, the family and the personal story of each individual – a sort of self-destruction involving a number of factors. These include oxidation processes particularly associated with free radicals;[1] a large auto-immunity process; hormonal and enzymatic disorders; and a subtle but systematic pathology in cerebral micro-circulation.

It is often too readily admitted that from a certain age, which varies according to the individual, there will automatically be a drop in the efficiency of cognitive mental activities – less creativity, a greater tendency towards mental fatigue, memory loss and, in particular, difficulties in forming, maintaining and recalling new memories, which, when associated with a weakening of central inhibition, explains why old people's 'present' tends to be invaded by old memories, not new. It is also more difficult to maintain delayed responses, and this, plus an inability to concentrate and a slower information processing, can be explained by a marked loss of neurons and their connections, particularly from the hippocampus and frontal areas.[2]

There is also a reduction in the brain's capacity to synthesise proteins and this also increases memory difficulties. From an electro-physiological point of view, alpha waves tend to slow down, there is decreased focusing and a

---

1 A molecule or atom disposing of a 'bachelor' electron on its external orbit. Usually in biology, one is dealing with an activated form of oxygen, strongly reacting with all surrounding molecules.

2 The frontal cortex is the anterior part of the cerebral cortex and is essentially implicated in short-term memory and in the programming feedback and control of complex behaviour. The hippocampus – a sub-cortical structure part of the limbic system – is implicated in long-term memory and emotional reactions.

general slowing down of EEG activity, and a reduction in the amount of paradoxical sleep, as well as a decrease in the amplitude of sensorial potentials in the cortex.[3] In addition to all this, the elderly tend to have more nervous breakdowns, less resistance to stress, increasing difficulty in changing habits and adapting to new situations and a marked reaction to the side-effects of medicines, etc.

Contrary to the unicist theories,[4] which were prevalent until some two or three years ago, it seems now that it is not only the cholinergic system which is deficient in the elderly, but in fact a whole set of systems. Taking account of large innate and acquired differences in individuals, the latest theory better explains the polymorphism of geropsychiatric symptoms.

The depressive tendency in the elderly is linked, for a great part, to a biological deficiency. With age, there is a significant increase in mono-amino-oxydase (MAO) activity (Robinson et al., 1972). Given the physiological role of MAO, of catabolizing mono-amines, including catecholamines and serotonine, i.e. the opposite action of anti-depressant drugs, it is understandable that this genetic order – to increase MAO activity with age – without being the only thing responsible, contributes to depression in the elderly.

It is clear then that there are many important symptoms associated with ageing. But I would like to put these a little in perspective on the basis of a number of experimental findings, and hope to show that

- deficiencies in the noetic (intellectual) sphere of old animals are linked to a number of factors, and that if we take all of these into account, an old animal can, within certain limits, behave like a young one;
- the environment, as a unified whole, can modify critically the noetic capacities not only of the young, but of the old.

Through a number of examples, I shall point to measures we can take to ensure the relatively normal functioning of the brain for as long as possible.

## *Long-term memory*

In traditional passive avoidance experiments on rats, the usual conclusion is that older animals remember unpleasant experiences (electric shocks) which they have associated with a certain place for a much shorter time than

---

[3] Impulses from all our sensory organs reach the cerebral cortex where they are decoded and give rise to perceptions.

[4] The unicist theories try to attribute cerebral age-related hypo-efficiency to one single deficiency, e.g. in the central cholinergic system which is the central nervous system synapses where the neuro-transmitter is acetyl-choline, a substance also important in the peripheral nervous system.

young ones and hence suffer more from memory deficiency (Kruse and Kohler, 1978). However, we have shown experimentally that the amount of deficiency is very variable and is much more nuanced depending on the conditions of the experiment (Soffié, 1987; Soffié and Giurgea, 1988).

For example, if the older rat is given an electric shock immediately upon entering a given place and hence associates more easily the two, it will remember this shock the next day and even twenty-nine days later. However, if the shock is given thirty seconds after it enters the given place, the older rat will remember the unpleasant experience much less well.

## *Behavioural rigidity*

It is fairly well known that elderly people have difficulty in adapting to new situations. Several studies have confirmed this tendency in experiments on rats and monkeys (Bartus et al., 1979). However, our studies have tended to show that such a deficiency in old rats is only apparent in certain well defined circumstances which very probably depend on the type of motivation involved (Soffié, 1987; Soffié and Giurgea, 1988).

In experiments where they had to learn an opposite tyoe of behaviour to one previously acquired, both young and old rats performed equally well when there was negative motivation, i.e. they received an electric shock when they did not choose the correct pathway in an experimental set-up. However, older rats performed much less well under positive motivation, i.e. they received peanuts for taking the correct pathway, which in this experimental set-up is a weaker motivation than the negative one, i.e. the painful electric shock.

There seems therefore to be behavioural rigidity only when the animals are positively motivated. We can put forward the hypothesis that with ageing there is a problem of cognitive effort linked to the type of motivation, and that this is the cause of the deficiency, and not a generalised and inexorable behavioural rigidity.

To extrapolate, we might say: if we motivate the elderly enough and give them the opportunity to do appropriate and interesting tasks, we will probably be surprised at how great their mental capacity can still be. We arrived at a similar conclusion after our third series of experiments.

## *Social memory*

Does an old rat recognise a young member of its own species? Experimentally we have found not only that an old or adult rat can easily distinguish between a young rat it has already met and one it has not, but that this older rat is curious and interested, particularly in a young rat it has never seen. We are a long way from the lack of curiosity and motivation shown in experiments where rats are presented with artificial stimuli (Brennan et al., 1984). It would appear then that older rats do not react in the same positive, interested way to artificial, non-alive, stimuli as they do to living members of their own species. Could we not extrapolate again about the need for human, social stimulation for the elderly?

## The geriatric vicious circle

Many studies have shown that socio-sensorial stimulation, handling and exercise can modify not only important cerebral parameters in older animals, but also, in certain cases, behavioural defects (Greenough, 1976). It has been proved that, in rats, a rich socio-sensorial environment both thickens the cerebral and pyriform cortex and significantly speeds up functional recovery from brain damage (Diamond et al., 1977).

There is therefore a great deal of experimental data on animals to help us reach a fundamental understanding of the so-called psycho-geriatric vicious circle (Lehmann, 1975). With age there is a decrease in RNA[5] and protein synthesis, a loss of neurotransmitters and neurons, and a drop in oxygen supply to the brain (of cardio-vascular and pulmonary origin and also due to lack of exercise, etc.)

These physiological factors bring about a drop in cognitive power and in turn add to and engender various social pressures (being taken out of the professional and economic cycle, family losses, etc.) creating negative and permanent emotional response. These in turn give rise to stress which, through a metabolic impact, reduces the metabolism and bloodflow of the brain and leads to an increase in cerebral hypoxia. This speeds up the rhythm of neuronal loss and gives rise to an increase in cognitive deficiency, which restarts and maintains the vicious circle.

We can use drugs at certain points in this cycle, not to 'get younger', but to slow the cycle down and so maintain efficient mental activity as long as possible. The importance of a rich socio-sensorial environment has already been mentioned, but it should be stressed again that by asking the elderly to do things, by requiring efforts of them that they can still make and which – deep down – they hope to be asked to make, their mood will be raised and they will once more feel useful. In this way they will fight against that depressive tendency which, encouraged by lack of motivation, reduces intellectual efficiency even further.

So a medical and drug-based approach to physiological cerebral ageing should also be accompanied by a psycho-social, environmental one, to ensure that the elderly can maintain an optimal level of cerebral activity

---

[5] Ribonucleic acid – an essential constituent of brain proteins.

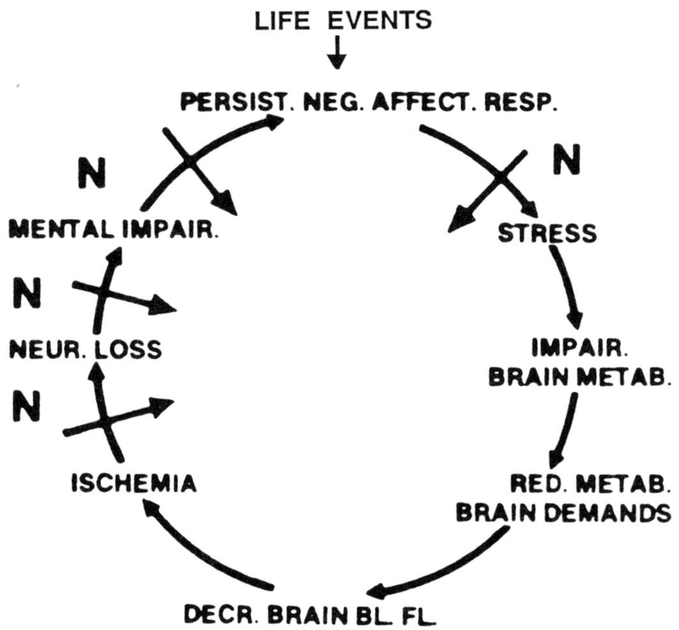


**Figure 14.1 Geropsychiatric Cycle (after Lehmann, 1975)**
**The elderly, due to various physiological and socio-economic factors, are prone to persistent negative emotional responses. These are sources of stress which in turn impair brain metabolism – usually through the reduction of cerebral metabolic demands – thus decreasing the basic blood flow. A certain degree of brain ischemia is therefore induced which accelerates neuronal loss and further aggravates mental impairment. Thus the self-perpetuating, deleterious vicious circle is maintained and continues.**

and continue to lead enjoyable and fulfilling lives, not only for themselves but for those around them. For, given the increasing number of elderly people in the world, it will be essential for society and humanity that older people play a more integrated and useful part as the years go on.

To paraphrase Sophocles: No one loves life as much as the old.

# References


Bartus, R.T., Dean, R.L. and Fleming, D.L., 'Aging in the Rhesus monkey: effects on visual discriminating learning and reversal learning', *J. Gerontol.*, vol. 34, no. 2, 1979, pp. 209–19.

Brennan, M.J., Allen, D., Aleman, D., Asmitia, E.C. and Quatermain, D., 'Age differences in within-session habituation of exploratory behaviour: effects of stimulus complexity', *Behavioral and Neural Biology*, no. 42, 1984, pp. 61–72.

Diamond, M.C., Johnson, R.E., Mizono, G., Stanley, I.P., Chong, L. Lee and Wells, M., 'Effects of Aging and Environment on the Pyroform Cortex, the Occipital Cortex and the Hippocampus', *Behav. Biology*, no. 20, 1977, pp. 325–36.

Domino, E.F., Dren, A.T. and Giardina, W.J., 'Biochemical and neurotransmitter changes in the aging brain,' in Lipton, Dimasco and Killam (eds), *Psychopharmacology. A Generation of Progress*, Raven Press, 1978, pp. 1507–15.

Greenough, W.T., 'Enduring Brain Effects of Differential Experience and Training', in Rosenzweig, M. and Bennett, E.L. (eds), *Neural Mechanisms of Learning and Memory*, MIT Press, 1976, pp. 255–78.

Kruse, H. and Kohler, H., 'Memory enhancing effects of piracetam in aged rats', *Fed. Proc. Pharmacol.*, vol. 37, no. 3548, 1978, p. 888.

Lehmann, H.E., 'Rational Pharmacotherapy in Geropsychiatry', 10th International Congress of Gerontology, Jerusalem, 22–27 June 1975, Abstract, pp. 22–23.

Robinson, D.S., Davis, J.M., Nies, A., Ravaris, C.L. and Sylvester, D., 'Relation of sex and aging to mono-amines oxydase activity of human brain, plasma and platelets, *Arch. Gen. Psychiatr.*, no. 24, 1972, pp. 536–9.

Soffié, M., 'Approche animale des modifications comportementales liées au vieillissement', *Bull. de la Classe des Sciences*, Acad. Royale de Belgique, series 5, vol. LXIII, no. 1, 1987, pp. 14–32.

Soffié, M. and Giurgea, C.E., 'Age-related memory impairments in rats: potential paradigms for pharmacological modulation', in Gruneberg, Morris and Sykes (eds), *Practical Aspects of Memory*, vol. 2, John Wiley and Sons, Chichester, 1988.

Chapter 15

# Mental health and the urban environment

by Hugh Freeman

Any one feature of the environment will have widely varying effects on the different people who may be exposed to it. These differing effects result from the variations in peoples' genetic constitutions and from the effect on them of their life experiences.

How can we analyse the environmental side – or input – of the equation, then? It consists of a series of signals which are received by the body and transmitted through psychological and physiological processes of enormous complexity. Such processes are mainly in the central nervous system and in the endocrine system, which are closely interrelated and have a common governing centre in the hypothalamus. Eventually, some of the environmental signals will be experienced as emotions. But the biological and psychological significance of these emotions will depend on various factors; these include an individual's culture and the way he has come to terms with his environment in the past.

Life experiences – probably through setting up conditioned reflexes – cause particular bodily organs to respond to environmental stimuli in particular ways; some of these will be maladaptive or harmful to the person concerned. Thus if three different people were exposed to the same environmental stress, they might show respectively a psychiatric disorder, a physical disorder or no ill effect at all. It is even possible for the stress to have a beneficial effect under certain conditions.

Our knowledge of the aetiology or causal chain of most psychiatric disorders is very incomplete. This is certainly true of environmental factors, as of other aspects. Therefore, any simplistic statement, such as 'bad housing causes mental illness', obviously cannot be correct because most people in bad housing do not become mentally ill. Situations which are as immensely complicated as this must never be approached from such a naïve position. Certain social situations may be coincident with a high rate of a particular form of morbidity, but scientifically, this allows us to say no more than that a connection between the two *could* exist.

Similarly, when considering any of the ecological studies of mental health, it is important to avoid the Ecological Fallacy: the assumption that trends which are based on averages for a geographical area can be applied to individuals living there. For instance, one area might have an excess of both schizophrenia and juvenile delinquency, but this does not mean that most delinquents are schizophrenic, or vice versa. Even if the two conditions did coexist in the same people, it would not necessarily be because of some common underlying process in the social structure.

## The psychological effects of the environment

The greatest unresolved problem in studying the psychological effects of the environment is to identify the processes of interaction between the social structure of a community and the individual's personality or behaviour. Community structure probably plays an important part in shaping individual values, attitudes, and behaviour; however, communities vary in their degree of integration, openness, etc. Deficiencies of social bonds are certainly a consequence of psychiatric illness, but failures of social networks may also be a factor increasing neurotic morbidity.

Stress is another concept that is very important in analysing the mediating processes between the environment and individual reactions. Stress can be seen primarily in physiological or psychological terms, and it is not clear which model is more crucial in determining human reactions. It has often been assumed that particular forms of stress (e.g. suppressed anger) would have causal relationships with specific clinical entities (e.g. hypertension), but this seems increasingly unlikely. Some people believe that social stress (e.g. poverty, stigmatisation, role disturbance from broken homes) are important aetiological factors in psychiatric disorder, but this has not really been proved.

A third important concept is information overload, which is particularly associated with the name of Stanley Milgram. This phenomenon is said to result from the man-made transformation of the physical environment and from the mass of symbols and messages produced by information technology. It accelerates both cultural change and shifts in value systems.

This in turn makes great demands on human adaptive capacity and may be concerned in the high mortality from diseases, such as coronary thrombosis, in developed societies.

It may well be that the ability of the human organism to process information is limited by its channel capacity. In that case, an excess of stimuli, relative to a person's processing capacity, would be a form of psycho-social stress. The coping strategies which may be used to escape from this situation – such as social withdrawal, use of drugs or psychiatric breakdown – are also likely to be harmful in themselves. Overload is relevant to social change because it is affected by time as well as by changes in absolute quantity. This model has an obvious significance for schizophrenia, which is believed to involve a constant state of over-arousal in the central nervous system.

Also important in schizophrenia is the 'Body Buffer Zone' – the characteristic distance which people keep between themselves and others – known also as 'personal space' or 'portable territory'. It is greater in schizophrenics than in normals, in introverts than in extroverts, and in violent prisoners than non-violent. Almost certainly, this is a protective mechanism against external stimuli to arousal. Since the extent of the 'zone' is purely subjective, it is governed both by culture and by personal characteristics of the individual.

Urban environments present us with physical and psychological stresses like high noise levels, crowding, relative anonimity, a high expectation of danger and anomie – the dissociation of social groups from guiding norms and the fragmentation of social groups, or 'social disintegration'. So far, there is little valid research to relate these stresses to specific forms of psychiatric disability, but our everyday experience confirms their unwelcome effects on us.

## Reducing over-arousal in urban environments

For the sake of both emotional and bodily health, it seems important, then, to reduce these states of constant over-arousal in the urban population. Fortunately, the human being is a very adaptable species and often finds ways of mitigating what would seem to be intolerable states of stress. But high arousal of the central nervous system is a very sinister process which does not cure itself by habituation. What, then, can be said about psychiatric disorder in relation to urbanisation generally?

In the world literature, there is a mountain of material on this subject, out of which you can get only a fair-sized mouse of firm conclusions. Studies from several countries have agreed that there are higher rates of identified psychiatric disorder in urban than in rural populations. But the word 'urban' may have different meanings in, say, Scandinavia, North America, or Asia, and it is still uncertain whether any true difference exists between urban and rural environments in levels of psychiatric morbidity.

Depression is essentially a social phenomenon, whose occurrence is highly related to the presence of three types of provoking agents:

- severe life events, mostly concerned with loss, e.g. arrangements for a new home falling through, or a job redundancy;
- major difficulties which last at least two years and do not concern health, e.g. poor housing (which was linked to 28 per cent of cases of chronic depression in a study by Brown and Harris);
- vulnerability factors, concerned with the support received from social relationships.

It is possible that the excess of depression which many researchers report in inner city women is related to lack of social support and lack of participation in a local community. These factors would be caused by high turnover of residents and changing ethnic composition, which tend to be found in such areas.

Turning to even milder and more common forms of psychiatric disorders, researchers find that the problems of identification and 'suburban neurosis' become almost overwhelming. The latter term was devised by Lord Taylor in 1938, from his experience as a doctor in a peripheral housing estate. He thought that the stresses involved in moving there from a central city area and living there resulted in a higher incidence of neurotic disturbances, particularly in women. Similarly, 'New Town Blues' has become a common cliché. So far, research has not provided any firm basis for this concept, though it seems that women generally do less well than men after such a move.

Hare and Shaw in a 1965 study of Croydon concluded that in any population there will be a vulnerable group whose health is below average, both mentally and physically, and which will tend to complain about its surroundings, largely as a projection of personal problems. Similarly, Taylor and Chave in 1964 concluded that about one-third of the adult population anywhere are troubled by at least some evidence of minor psychiatric ill health.

With children, though, the situation may be somewhat different. Rutter and Quinton compared a group of 10-year-olds in an inner London borough with children of the same age in the Isle of Wight and found that emotional disorders, conduct disorders and specific reading retardation were all twice as common in the city group. In both areas, child disorder and deviance were found to be associated with four variables: family discord, parental deviance, social disadvantage, and adverse school characteristics. These features were very significantly more common in London: thus there appear to be forces in the life of the inner city which predispose to the development of mental health problems in children. But it is not yet possible to say exactly what these environmental problems are.

## *The effects of architecture*

Social change, which includes migration and rehousing, will have the greatest impact where there is a marked contrast between the family's previous social context and that which it finds in the new community. Such a contrast is most likely to occur when the family comes from an old, stable, working-class neighbourhood, such as Bethnal Green in London, or the West End of Boston. These were close-knit communities, based on long residence and intermarriage, where social groups were centred on a familiar physical environment with many informal meeting places. They were also characterised by an intermingling of the buildings of home and work – something which planners have perhaps reacted against too strongly.

The United Kingdom has carried out an enormous relocation of people from the old communities which were the products of the Industrial Revolution. But the only real study of the emotional impact of such migration is American and was published by Fried in 1963. Among the former inhabitants of a slum area of Boston, nearly half the women felt sad and depressed for at least six months and more than a quarter felt the same two years after moving. The proportion of men showing long-term grief reactions was only slightly smaller; in addition, there were many other people of both sexes who were troubled by less severe depressive feelings.

Fried points out that in this type of community, the local area around the dwelling unit is seen as an integral part of home and contains interlocking sets of social networks. Breaking up the external basis for interpersonal and communal relationships destroys the sense of group identity of many people, which is bound up with their sense of spatial identity. The result is a deep experience of loss; with some justice, Fried called his study 'Grieving for a Lost Home.'

This leads on to the question of so-called 'comprehensive urban redevelopment' and its undoubtedly disastrous effects. There has been no scientific investigation of the harm suffered by individuals and communities from this policy of bulldozing everything above ground level. Human feelings have been ruthlessly trampled on by these urban clearances; in clinical practice I hear all too often from patients about the ill effects that have resulted.

Peter Willmott has pointed out that the whole process of redevelopment can take as long as ten years, during which time people are worried about their future, watch the decay of the neighbourhood around them, and may finally be moved against their will. As Gans has emphasised, clearance destroys not only buildings, but functioning social systems. On the other hand, if people can stay in or near their old homes, communities remain stable and their informal networks of advice and assistance result in fewer demands on public services. This self-help can never be artificially reproduced.

Public housing policy is far too monolithic in its ideas and in the way it operates. One of the most bizarre examples of this was the high-rise fashion – enthusiastically embraced by architects and developers and supported by government subsidies. It failed to achieve any of the advantages that were claimed, and its adverse human and social consequences – particularly for families with young children – are probably a permanent fact of life now. It would have been better to have examined these consequences before the policy was generally applied, rather than afterwards.

High-rise living is particularly hard on those who are below average in social assets, since the support they might expect in traditional neighbourhoods is lost. These people are also likely to have difficulty in coping with the more complex aspects of a high-technology environment, particularly when these start going wrong – and they invariably *do* go wrong, because public housing authorities never have the resources for proper maintenance of these structures.

There is a need to conserve – or to provide again in the many places where it has been lost – the social matrix in which a worthwhile quality of life and work can grow. If we use our technological knowledge to serve us, rather than to destroy us, it is possible to create a milieu which is both efficient and human. It is also possible to preserve the identity of places, rather than turning the whole country into a Nowheresville of uniform concrete and plastic. This is not just impractical folksiness. By such redevelopment we have been progressively wiping out the collective memory of our cities and towns. Continuity is an essential requirement for psychological health, and this unprecedented scale and speed of change could well be a recipe for social disaster.

It seems very foolhardy to discard features of the environment which have grown up over centuries. Marks has examined the ethological background to agoraphobia – the morbid dread of public places or open spaces: he has shown that this disorder may involve opto-kinetic reflexes concerned in space and light perception. Agoraphobics often feel easier in the dark and better in winter than in summer; many people feel uncomfortable next to a high window or a wall of glass. These biological considerations suggest that there may well be advantages to mental health in more traditional forms of living arrangement – for instance, a terraced street or court.

The sheer size of today's urban settlements also involve a considerable psychological problem. The great cities of the past were quite small by our standards, but megalopolises like Tokyo or the US eastern seaboard result in what Cappon has called 'the destruction of whatever natural order of territoriality was established by historical and social usage'. Since identity of person seems to have a great deal to do with identity of place, there is likely to be much danger to psychological health from the incomprehensible size of present-day urban areas, their severance by dangerous polluting motorways, and the monotony of tower blocks separated by hostile, impersonal spaces.

Terence Lee has shown that people see the environment in terms of socio-spatial schemata, which are related to prominent boundaries and areas of ground, rather than to density or to population numbers. Density in itself has not been shown to have any adverse effects, so that while we need not be afraid of high density, we should respect those boundary markings.

There is an urgent need for psychological conservation areas, just as there is for physical conservation areas – a need to restore the benefits of urbanity. That means the diversity of choices, the chances for accidental encounters to occur, all within an identifiable area: the essential qualities of good communities in the past.

Such socio-cultural disintegration must surely have adverse psychological effects on people. But much more serious study of the relationship between the environment and mental health is required if the political process is to be influenced.

One particular contribution which social psychiatry might make is to oppose the overwhelming preoccupation that planners, architects, and local governments have had for many years with reduction of urban density. Relatively high density is actually essential for the positive qualities of towns and cities, such as cultural life and specialised professional services. However, up to now, attempts to apply psychiatric knowledge to the social field have tended to be focused at far too ambitious a level. The use of established knowledge could now reduce a number of forms of psychiatric and social pathology, in modest but worthwhile ways. In the long run, though, progress can only come through scrupulous research, based on clearly defined concepts, and through action which is directly related to what has been scientifically demonstrated.

# References


Brown, G.W. and Harris, T., *Social Origins of Depression*, Tavistock, London, 1978.

Cappon, D., 'Designs for improvements in the quality of life in downtown cases', *International Journal of Mental Health*, no. 4, 1975, pp. 31–47.

Fried, M., 'Grieving for a lost home', in Duhl, L.J. (ed.), *The Urban Condition*, Basic Books, New York, 1963.

Hare, E.H. and Shaw, G.K., *Mental Health on a New Housing Estate*, Oxford University Press, London, 1965.

Lee, T., *Psychology and the Environment*, Methuen, London, 1976.

Marks, I.M., *Fears and Phobias*, Heinemann, London, 1969.

Rutter, M.L. and Quinton, D., 'Psychiatric disorder – ecological factors and concepts of causation', in McGurk, H. (ed.), *Ecological Factors in Human Development*, North Holland, Amsterdam, 1977.

Taylor, S., 'Suburban Neurosis', *Lancet*, no. 1, 1988, pp. 759–61.

Taylor, S. and Chave, S.P.W., *Mental Health and Environment*, Longman, London, 1964.

Willmott, P., 'Population and Community in London', *New Society*, no. 30, 1974, pp. 206–9.

Chapter 16

# Housing and the home after 150 years of industrial society

by F.W. Häussler

One hundred and fifty years of industrialization have wrought profound technological and social change in our society. Actions based on new views about economics and culture have affected natural systems and unbalanced our environment. Even the construction and design of buildings is bound up with the severe stresses of life today.

The early years of the century and, again, the past thirty years saw a boom in housing construction which has been a technical revolution in itself. An array of new materials has opened hitherto undreamed-of vistas and opportunities in the building world. But in the flush of progress we have tended to forget that our homes, their surroundings and, indeed, the environment itself should reflect these drastic changes in the way we live. After all, they affect our physical and mental well-being, the way we think and behave, our very health itself.

To blame, no doubt, is the lack of understanding of the spiritual and psychological changes in people over the last one hundred and fifty years, changes which have often been in marked contrast to sweeping technological development. It would not matter that we roam space and split the atom if only our minds had been able to keep up with our own technological sophistication, if the human measure had retained its full sway.

### *The home as a source of environmental stress*

Human beings need sunlight, air and green spaces in order to flourish. But very little thought has so far been given to the actual 'four-walls-and-a-roof' of housing – our most intimate environment – which we need in order to feel safe in our industrialized, mass culture society. Structural changes have occurred which in no way reflect our domestic habits. *Residential sociology* – the science of human behaviour in the home environment – has shown that while people apparently blithely accept the accomplishments of the age, they really have very little understanding of the laws of the technological universe and tend to underestimate the dangers it may present.

Unfortunately, technological progress can be inimical to human health, not only through the grand ramifications of societal development but also through such 'small' matters as its impacts on housing design. It is not easy to overlook the exceptional, but far too easy to be blind to the ordinary things in life. Yet the humdrum facts of the daily round form the fabric of the life we must hand on.

For example, we take for granted the ordinary things of day-to-day living – electric light, piped hot water, the dishwasher, the telephone, the vacuum cleaner, the automobile, typewriters and pocket calculators. We even take computers in our stride, although we do not know how the energy they consume is generated or whether they are as safe as they appear! We are, in fact, only just beginning to ask questions and to turn to science for answers which are still a long way off.

We are talking about the quality of life and the home as they relate to human health. We have neglected the human factor, as opposed to technical development, for so long that our homes have actually become a source of injury without our realising it.

## What is a home?

Our homes are the centre of our lives, the nest we need to renew ourselves. A home is a secure haven of return, a place of peace to offset the agitation of the outside world. Remember, the wider community stands or falls with the quality of its homes. Our home and family are the source of regeneration and will help to provide answers even to the burning issues of our time. Learning to recognise and appreciate the psychological, health and technical dimensions of 'living at home' is vital to a liveable future.

The trouble is that the space designed in modern housing has not been adapted to suit people. Rather, it is people who have been expected to adapt to what has been on offer. Until very recently, little effort was made to find out whether the new materials and techniques – e.g. heating, thermal insulation, picture windows, concrete structures, etc. – are really 'good' for people or whether any inherent faults might be corrected before the dwellings are completed. Likewise, little attempt was made to analyse modern living conditions before or after the construction of housing blocks.

So, technical advances combined with ignorance about their impacts is the explanation of why our residential structures in cities and in rural areas are ill-designed and why we suffer stress just from living in 'modern' surroundings.

### *Designing homes as shelters*

Traffic, especially private transport, is a problem. Individual mobility is very much a product of industrialization. The endless tailbacks on our weekend motorways and gridlocked city streets are not a harmonious way of life and they lead to feelings of unrest and dissipation. A well-balanced home environment could compensate for external cacophony. But, unfortunately, few so-called modern dwellings are designed and appointed to nurture the spirit, to give the 'shelter' we know we need. The outside world is not excluded from our homes, and so we flee our homes to go anywhere, no matter where, *else*where.

### *Designing homes for changing families*

Industrialization has also changed the structure of the family, but this phenomenon is not reflected in the construction of housing. We must think of ways to build homes that are 'family-friendly'. We need houses that can grow with a young family and shrink as growing children leave home. We need houses which can welcome the return of grandparents when the children have left the nest.

The elderly should be allowed to live in the socially dynamic family environment. Homes for the elderly should be the exception, not the rule. Older people should not be rejected, but welcomed and allowed to be socially useful by carrying out the tasks which suit their years and which give them pleasure, such as looking after their grandchildren.

In particular, we need houses which can accommodate the changing roles of men and women in the home as in society. Now that most women work outside the house, families are making different demands on their houses. Even the most rabid feminists will have to agree that 'housework' is not slavery but an important *job in the home.* Families and babies are not really the secondary concerns they appear to have become in industrialized society. They may change a woman's professional life and her development, but they do *not* block them. Our dwellings should reflect these changing attitudes.

### *Building homes for families*

Can we build such houses? Are there models or principles we can apply to the empty shell, so that people of all persuasions, lifestyles, opinions can develop a personal way of living in them – apart from the aspect of interior decoration?

The answer is, yes, we can. We have not seen much of it yet – the headlong pursuit of individual, material well-being has prevented us from doing so, in part because after the devastation of the cities in the Second World War people increasingly lost their awareness of the wider community.

We can build family-friendly dwellings if we keep in mind two important principles. First, interior space should be fluid and flexible. For example, a design is flexible when it offers modifiable floorspace, interchangeable rooms, and the possibility of changing the number of rooms. Second, the (preferably open-plan) kitchen should be the centre of family life. The kitchen, the hearth, is the place where families meet to eat, to talk, and even to think. It is a place of communion, a place to nourish not only the body but the family spirit as well.

How is the family-friendly home to be built? By means of new construction or restoration? For planners, this is a question of setting public and private priorities. For the inhabitants it is a learning process. There are three areas where priorities must be set:

- communicability
- privacy
- functionality.

The family-friendly solutions offer alternatives to the straitjacket of European thinking about residential architecture which tended to insist on building with fixed, usually load-bearing walls, meaning an inflexible use of the total space in the dwelling. However, this is the technical aspect of the matter, and technical solutions are thirteen to the dozen.

To summarise, people cannot really keep pace with technological progress. There is also a limit to what we can cope with in technical and material output. When we say progress, then we really should mean research – to see whether the plunge into the unknown is justified and what its impacts on us may be.

## Educating people about the home

The problems outlined above and their repercussions on residential and town planning can only be tackled at the source. People must be brought up from an early age to see connections, learn about context.

The real crux will be to get the politicians and society to recognise that the domestic environment should also be part of the educational curriculum. At the moment, much of what we believe about the domestic environment comes to us unawares and much of what we learn in this way may be wrong.

Education of children and adolescents about the domestic environment will prove to be just as important as the question of whether old, dependent people can return to the family circle without disrupting the flow of family life. We shall need time to do this. And we shall need to exchange experience and knowledge across the continents.

Technological progress brings us closer together, not only in space but also in attitudes. But nature and human nature are the counterpart of technical progress and they will not be forgotten. Technical progress must adjust to nature, not the other way round. It is not real progress and must not be allowed to rule over nature and the human race. We have unshackled and developed untold technological forces – now we must accept our responsibilities, and these include an area which we have always taken too much for granted: our homes.

Chapter 17

# Ecological principles in town planning: the impact of vegetation on the quality of life in the city

by Aloys Bernatzky

On 9 June 1987 the German Press Agency (dpa) dispatched the following news item from New York:

> **Half the world's population to become city dwellers by the year 2000?**
>
> The number of people living in large urban concentrations is growing steadily, especially in the developing countries. By the turn of the century, over 50% of the world population will live in cities. UN population statistics now indicate that roughly two billion people (42% of the world population) were city dwellers in 1985, as against some 3 billion living in rural areas. The UN experts predict that the world's urban population will have grown to 3.7 billion by the year 2010.
>
> The same survey indicates that there were 99 cities in 1985 with more than 2 million inhabitants. Twelve of these – eight in developing countries, four in the industrialized world – contained more than 10 million souls. UN experts reckon that there will be 23 cities over 10 million by the year 2000, of which 17 will be located in less-developed countries.

As cities rapidly increase in size, we can expect the natural urban climate to degenerate proportionately. Restoring natural living conditions will be our only option to counter this trend and our only ally in this work will be urban vegetation – green areas and trees – in the right places. Correctly planned, this can provide many benefits.

## Air purification

We know from studies carried out throughout the world that green areas and trees can cleanse the air of dust and chemical pollutants. Trees and large shrubs inhibit the load capacity of air, causing solid air pollutants to form sediments.

**Table 17.1.**
**Control of particulates from vegetation in Frankfurt am Main, FRG**
*(particles/litre of air)*

| Location | morning | afternoon | evening |
|---|---|---|---|
| Main railway station | 16,380 | 18,310 | 17,640 |
| City centre | 15,120 | 13,220 | 18,370 |
| Streets without trees | 12,880 | 10,180 | 11,490 |
| Streets with trees | 3,870 | 3,040 | 3,830 |
| Park | 3,260 | 1,180 | 3,140 |

Source: W. Lamp, 1947

In tree-filled parks, up to eighty-five per cent of suspended particulates may be filtered out; trees planted along streets may reduce particulates by up to seventy per cent, assuming that they have been correctly planted and spaced: close enough, yet not too close. Even naked trees in winter still perform at about sixty per cent of the summer rate. In addition, trees lining urban streets can filter out a substantial proportion of lead particulates from automobile exhaust (Keller, 1974).

## Temperature reduction

The only way to keep cities from overheating is to maintain unbuilt open areas planted with grass and trees. Even the 50–100 metre green strip on the traffic ring around the city centre in Frankfurt has brought about a drop in temperature of up to 3.5° C on hot summer days, as much as though the city were at an altitude of + 700 metres.

Much depends on the kind of vegetation planted. In the daytime, the cooling effect of tree-grown spaces in the city is considerable, since trees provide more leaf coverage than any other plant occupying the same space.

**Table 17.2**
**The impact of trees on the thermal balance**

| | |
|---|---|
| Rainwater run-off in areas covered by vegetation: (The remainder evaporates or is absorbed into the soil) | 5–15 per cent |
| Run-off in cities lacking vegetation: (This is carried off by the drains and is therefore not available for evaporation) | approx. 60 per cent |
| At an average rainfall of 600 mm/year this represents: | 360 $mm/m^2$ = 360 $litres/m^2$ or 3,600 $m^3$/hectare |

Source: Bernatzky, 1978.

Lawns, on the other hand, can get quite hot very quickly in the daytime, so that grassy spaces around high-rise concrete apartment blocks provide virtually no cooling effect whatsoever. Their slight cooling effect is offset, in fact overwhelmed, by the heat accumulating effect of the buildings. The same goes for the newly popular roof plantings, which tend to be grass anyway.

At night, however, the roles are reversed. Temperatures above lawns, meadows and fields drop dramatically, releasing cool air which, if the topographical conditions are right, flows into neighbouring built-up areas. Tree-filled areas, on the other hand, are warmer than open areas because the heat is trapped by the trees.

How does this cooling effect come about? Vegetation, owing to its low mass, stores little or no heat at all, so that a radiation balance is quickly achieved in green areas. Plants reflect the most radiation; some sixty to seventy-five per cent of the radiation absorbed is used to evaporate the moisture which the plant had taken up from the soil.

Table 17.2 represents an annual water consumption of 360 trees, i.e. an annual consumption of 10 $m^3$/tree. If there are no trees, 3,600 $m^3$/ha of rainfall will disappear into the drains and be lost to evaporation. The city is then left with $2.16 \times 10^9$ kilocalories (kcal) of heat from solar radiation, which, when added to man-made heat from a variety of incineration processes, can cause overheating: virtual heat islands throughout the city. Turning the equation around, we can conclude that 360 trees generate a cooling power of $2.16 \times 10^9$ kcal/ha/per annum. In contrast, popular, easy-care green spaces made of careful selections of potted plants ('architects' parsley') set out in public squares and places generate no cooling effect at all.

In contrast, a city which lacks vegetation stores excess warmth in the layers of air closest to the ground and buildings, which at night radiate back the heat that had been absorbed during the day, giving rise to the well-known urban 'oven heat' phenomenon.

### *Local winds bring fresh air to the city*

Local winds can improve the air supply in cities in several ways: from winds along the earth's surface ('field winds') drawn by barometric 'lows' in the inner cities, and from descending flows of cold air from neighbouring slopes at night. The air must flow over or through vegetation, and these two possibilities can mutually reinforce each other. When these processes are at work, even a single tree can become a cooling unit. Urban aeration can also be fostered by restoring canalised, i.e. covered, brooks and streams in built-up areas to their natural state. Opening up these waterways and restoring the vegetation on their banks will improve the appearance of the city as well as generating and reinforcing all the effects of green areas mentioned so far: air purification, cooling and aeration.

## Noise abatement

Plants can help to reduce noise in urban areas by up to 12 decibels, as Table 17.3 shows. All the shrubs and trees listed can help to reduce noise in the frequency bands between 1,000 and 11,200 Hertz (Hz), the best band being 8,000 Hz. However, they must have foliage right to the very ground. Conifers are not quite so effective.

**Table 17.3**
**Noise abatement**

| 4–6 decibels | 6–8 decibels | 8–10 decibels | 10–12 decibels |
|---|---|---|---|
| *Juniperus chinensis 'Pflitzeriana'* | *Carpinus betulus* | *Populus x berolinensis* | *Acer pseudoplatanus* |
| *Alnus incana* | *Fagus sylvatica* | *Tilia platyphyllus* | |
| *Acer negundo* | *Ilex aquifolium* | *Viburnum lantana* | |
| *Betula pendula* | *Philadelphus pubescens* | *Viburnum rhytidophyllum* | |
| *Cornus sanguinea* and *alba* | *Quercus robur* | | |
| *Corylus avellana* | *Rhododendron* | | |
| *Crataegus prunifolia* | *Syringa vulgaris* | | |
| *Forsythia x intermedia* | | | |
| *Lonicera mackii* and *L. ledebouri* | | | |
| *Populus canadensis*, hybrids | | | |
| *Sambucus nigra* | | | |
| *Tilia cordata* | | | |

Source: Beck, 1967.

**Table 17.4**
**Oxygen values in Frankfurt am Main**

| | |
|---|---|
| In the Palm Garden Park | 18.5 vol.% |
| in the neighbouring streets | 17.0 vol.% |
| in the vicinity of the town hall | 16.8 vol.% |
| in the city centre | 17.0 vol.% |

Source: Bernatzky, unpublished.

## The contribution of trees to the oxygen supply

The atmosphere is said to contain so much $O_2$ that we need not fear it will run out. This is only partly true. Oxygen production and consumption via biological processes have so far remained in equilibrium, in fact with a slight superiority on the production side. Now that we are burning increasing quantities of fossil fuels and clearing more forest lands we are using up vast quantities of oxygen. Five billion tonnes of $CO_2$ produced by fossil fuel

**Table 17.5**
**Oxygen production by various ecosystems**

| **Ecosystem** | **Area** ($10^6$ km$^2$) | **$O_2$ production** (t/ha/yr) | **Total $O_2$** ($10^9$ t/yr) |
|---|---|---|---|
| *Forest* | | | |
| Temperate cold-foliage | 8 | 26.0 | 20.8 |
| Boreal-mixed conifer | 15 | 15.6 | 23.4 |
| Temperate rain forest | 1 | 31.2 | 3.1 |
| Tropical & sub-tropical rain forest | 10 | 39.0 | 39.0 |
| Miscellaneous dry forest | 14 | 5.2 | 7.3 |
| **Sub-total** | **48** | **117.0** | **93.6** |
| *Non-forest* | | | |
| Agriculture | 15 | 10.4 | 15.6 |
| Meadows and grassland | 26 | 7.8 | 20.3 |
| Tundra-type | 12 | 2.6 | 3.1 |
| Other wilderness | 32 | 2.6 | 8.3 |
| Frozen wastes (ice) | 15 | - | - |
| **Sub-total** | **100** | **23.4** | **47.3** |
| **Continents** | **148** | **147.4** | **140.9** |

Sources: Reichle, 1970, and Hansen, 1975.

incineration and another five billion tonnes of $CO_2$ resulting from forest clearings (land clearing, increased rates of humus oxidation) are released into the atmosphere each year (Woodwill, 1979). These ten billion tonnes of $CO_2$ correspond to the consumption of around eight billion tonnes of oxygen. These figures apply to oxygen consumption in the bottom layers of the atmosphere which provide the air which people breathe. Table 17.4 shows oxygen values which the author found at the end of September 1978 in the air in Frankfurt on a rainy day with a stiff west wind blowing.

In the absence of windy weather, the oxygen shortage in city centres can only be compensated for by the presence of vegetation. Under these circumstances, green areas and trees are a kind of emergency oxygen tank (Tables 17.5 and 17.6).

**Table 17.6**
**Oxygen production by type of tree**

| Species | t/h/yr |
|---|---|
| Birch | 9.5 |
| Beech | 15.6 |
| Oak | 11.5 |
| Larch | 15.6 |
| Douglas Fir | 19.3 |
| Fir | 15.6 |
| Pine | 10.3 |

Sources: Polster, 1950, and Hansen, 1975.

In 1971, F. Davitaya said: ' ... if the annual decrease [in oxygen] continues at 10 billion tonnes, we can expect two thirds of the total free oxygen supply in the atmosphere and the hydrosphere to run out in 100,000 years and we must then expect carbon dioxide levels in the atmosphere to reach danger point. In actual fact, however, both oxygen consumption and carbon dioxide levels will continue to rise. An annual increase of one per cent will take us to critical levels in only 700 years, with a five per cent upturn it will take us 180 years and a ten per cent rise will leave us with a critical build-up in just 100 years.' Needless to say, no city has enough vegetation to produce the quantities of oxygen needed to offset the amounts consumed. But that does not entitle us to ignore the evidence. Fifty years ago we thought we had enough pure water to last forever; our belief in unlimited oxygen resources may prove equally false. So what can be undertaken to correct this trend?

Trees and green areas are important for relaxation and recreation. The average citizen spends ten per cent of net leisure time on an annual holiday, twenty per cent of net leisure time at the weekend, and seventy per cent of net leisure time at home. That means that green spaces are needed close by (for example, at walking and baby stroller distance).

Furthermore, well-planted green areas between buildings can provide inhabitants with a private lifeline. Where homes are open to the outside world on the street side, they should be equally open at the back with a green road for pedestrians and children connecting the tracts of land. This way inhabitants can spend more time out of doors.

Of course we must make sure that all pre-conditions are met so that the green spaces can function optimally: this includes the very best ecological bases and thorough knowledge of biological, ecological and meteorological prerequisites

There is no such thing as passive green! Even if nobody were to visit them, the green areas would still fulfil their climate-conditioning function.

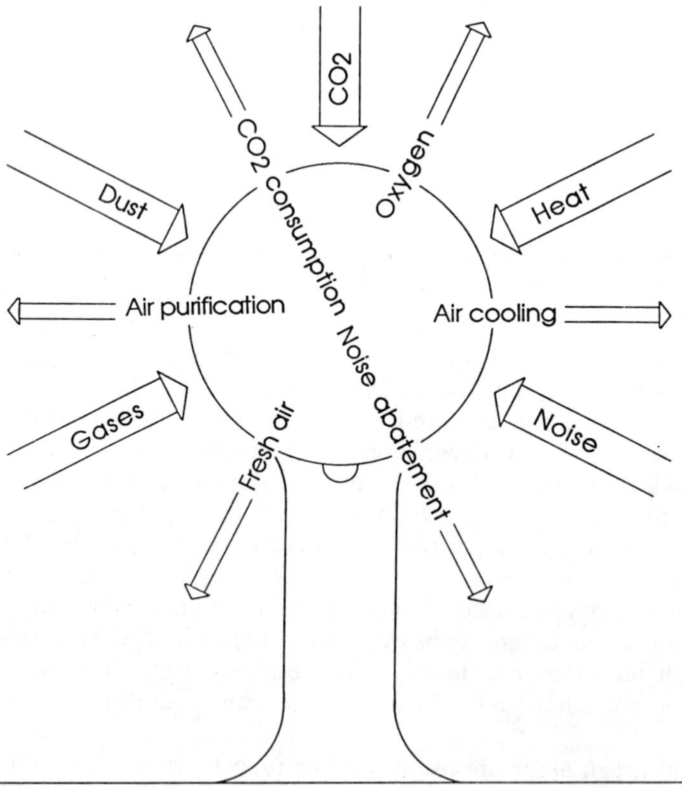


**Figure 17.1 The environmental functions of a tree**

## Caring for the city's lungs

But there are trees and trees! What matters is not so much how many trees a city has, but rather how much foliage these trees have. Urban trees tend to be diseased, not, generally speaking, because of air pollution but because the ecological conditions for their growth are inadequate: their roots are increasingly sealed off, the soil gradually becomes compressed and generally lacks sufficient air, water and nutrients. Another sore point is the way in which the trees are cared for; a tree which has its crown cut back cannot fulfil its environmental function for city dwellers. Only whole and healthy trees will do (Table 17.7).

Lastly, although the well-planted median strips on our motorways and roads look very nice, their contribution to urban hygiene is nil! It would be much better to forget about planting trees on the median strips, and instead to build wider pavements and plant trees there, keeping in mind that isolated plants in tubs or boxes will not do the job.

Look at the difference in the quality of urban life in a bare city as opposed to one with trees:

| Without trees | With trees |
|---|---|
| High dust levels | Air purification |
| Overheating | Air cooling |
| Dry air | Increase in relative atmospheric humidity |
| Stagnant air | Aeration |
| Gaseous air pollution | $CO_2$ consumption/oxygen production |
| Inhuman/denatured city | Spiritually/physically healthy city |

It is not the fault of existing urban green areas that they are not as effective as they might be. It is the fault of poor, arbitrary designs and distribution of vegetation and green areas within the city which is to blame. Town planners and landscape architects need to develop new approaches to the use of vegetation in the city.

The environmental value of green areas can be summarised as follows:

- *Air cooling by evaporation:* up to 3.5° C/100 metre-wide plantation (in Frankfurt), depending on leaf surface area and location of the plantation;
- *Generation of cold air:* resulting in fresh air supply, aeration of the city;
- *Air purification:* in parks up to eighty-five per cent; in treelined streets up to seventy per cent; in winter (no leaves) up to sixty per cent of the above values;
- *Oxygen production:* 600 kg$O_2$/ha of green area/12 hours, at 900 kg $CO_2$ consumption;
- *Noise abatement:* through wood planting (up to 12 dB, depending on the type of wood/shrub and on the spacing).

**Table 17.7**

**Functional value of a 100-year-old beech tree standing by itself in optimal ecological conditions [a]**

| | |
|---|---|
| **Dimensions of the tree** | |
| Height | 25 m |
| Crown span | 14 m |
| Crown volume | 2,700 $m^3$ |
| Surface area | 160 $m^2$ |
| Outer leaf surface | 1,600 $m^2$ |
| Interior leaf area | 160,000 $m^2$ |
| (total intercellular partitions) | |
| Wood mass | 15 $m^3$ |
| Dry weight | 12,000 kg |
| of which pure carbon | 6,000 kg |
| **Physiological functions** | |
| Water absorption | 0.960 kg/h |
| $CO_2$ absorption | 2.352 kg/h |
| Oxygen production | 1.712 kg/h[b] |
| Glucose production | 1.600 kg/h |
| Total evaporation | 10 $m^3$/Joule[c] |
| **Psychological functions** | |
| Fundamental experience of nature | |
| Environmental exchange | |
| Tranquillising hues | |
| Oasis of peace | |
| Natural rhythm | |
| Spiritual restoration/relaxation | |

[a] This tree produces a year's supply of oxygen for ten people; 150 $m^2$ leaf surface area generates enough oxygen for one person per year, according to Heinrich Walter, Grundlagen des Pflanzenlebens, 1950, p. 171.

[b] It would take 5,400 young trees with a crown volume of 0.5 $m^3$ to maintain the function of this beech tree.

[c] = heat consumption of $8.10^6$/kcal/Joule.

Source: A. Bernatzky, 1978 a.

It is clear that green areas composed of trees and other vegetation can help to compensate for much of the damage done by unnatural (denatured) urban construction to the climate. The implications of this for our physical and spiritual/psychological health are legion. We also find here an answer to the question how 'naturally' people should live, how 'humane' their living environment ought to be – an answer devoid of ideological or other bias.

# References


Beck, G., *Pflanzen als Mittel der Lärmbekämpfung*, 1967.

Bernatzky, A., *Von der mittelalterlichen Stadtbefestigung zu den Wallgrünflächen von Heute. A contribution to the issue of green spaces in German towns*, 1960.

Bernatzky, A., 'Die Bedeutung von Schutzplanzungen gegen Luftverunreinigungen', Air pollution proceedings of the first European Congress on the Influence of Air Pollution on Plants and Animals, Wageningen, 1968, pp. 383–395.

Bernatzky, A., *Tree ecology and preservation*, 1978a.

Bernatzky, A., 'Bäume in der Stadt – "Architekten-Petersilie" oder "Grüne Lunge?"', *Bild der Wissenschaft*, vol. 11, 1978b, pp. 144–58.

Davitaya, F., 'Verschmutzung der Erdatmosphäre und Veränderung ihrer Gaszusammensetzung', Izv. Akad. Nauk. SSSR (Rep. Acad. Sci. Soviet Socialist Republics, Geogr. series N° 4); German summary in *Ideen des exakten Wissens*, 1971.

Hansen, H.H., *Die Pflanze als Sauerstofflieferant*, biology-botany exam paper, University of Saarland, 1975.

Keller, T., 'Die Sauerstoffbilanz der Schweiz', *Schweiz. Zeitschrift Forstwesen*, no. 124, 1973, pp. 465–73.

Lamp, W., *Untersuchungen über den Staubgehalt einer vom Krieg teilweise zerstörten Grossstadt*, Examination paper, Darmstadt Polytechnic, Darmstadt, 1947.

Landsberg, 'Micrometeorological Temperature Differentiation through Urbanisation', *Urban Climate*, WMO techn. note no. 108, 1970, pp. 129–36.

Polster, H., *Die Physiologischen Grundlagen der Stofferzeugung im Walde. Untersuchungen über Assimilation, Respiration und Transpiration unserer Hauptholzarten, 1950.*

Reichle, D.E., 'Analysis of temperate forest ecosystems', *Ecological Studies*, vol. 2, 1970.

Sukopp, H., et al., *Ökologisches Gutachten über die Auswirkungen von Bau und Betrieb der BAB Berlin West auf den grossen Tiergarten.*

Walter, H., *Einführung in die Phytologie I, Grundlagen des Pflanzenlebens*, 1950.

Woodwell, G.M., 'Das Kohlendioxidproblem', *Spektrum der Wissenschaft*, vol. 1, 1950, pp. 11–18.

Chapter 18

# The crisis in industrial societies at the dawn of the 21st century

by Jean-Marie Pelt

This chapter could have been entitled 'Putting an end to the nineteenth century' because we are witnessing the death today of much that was born then:

- ideologies: liberalism, socialism and Marxism;
- the industrial revolution, which modified social conditions totally over the planet;
- a blind belief in progress engendered by the tremendous development of science.

## Malthus, Darwin and Marx

In the late eighteenth century, Malthus put forward the claim that the first law of the newly developing economics was the law of the strongest – when populations grow and resources do not, it is the poor who are the first hit.

Darwin applied to nature what Malthus had done for human society. It was the struggle for survival, the selection of the fittest or best which made species evolve from age to age. But he was talking about geological ages on the surface of the earth.

Marx applied Darwin's ideas to the social conditions created by the first industrial revolution. The struggle for survival became the struggle between classes. Evolutionary laws explained the meaning of history. Just as mammals had succeeded reptiles and batrachians, and flowering plants ferns and moss, so would a new social class succeed feudal and bourgeois dominance. The proletarian dictatorship was born.

Political systems grew out of these new ideologies. In the twentieth century, liberalism – based on free competition and the survival of the fittest individuals – fought constantly against variations of socialism and Marxism – based on the struggle between classes. In the middle of all this, and in the political centre, social democrats and Christian democrats in Europe tried to survive as well as they could in the stifling ideological climate of perpetual class struggle. As the twentieth century moves to its close, politicians and citizens from all political parties are still fighting for their place in the sun.

But I believe that these bitter struggles are in fact only the external manifestation of the underlying desire for power of the ego, of the 'I'. For the average citizen nineteenth century ideologies became identified as: 'Marxism is others working for me – and good for me. Liberalism is me working for me – and too bad for the others.' Both liberalism – based on unrestrained competition (me first) – and Marxism – based on class struggle (us alone) – are declining in Europe. And as they die we are perceiving one of the fundamental biological truths of our primate brains – that we need constantly to engage in struggles for power. This is really and only what political organisations want and do. The ideologies of the last century have dressed up and painted over this truth most skilfully. As they decline, people will see this more and more clearly.

## A new type of society

After the industrial revolution in all its successive variations, then the industrial society, we are now entering the post-industrial society – the hi-tech or communication society.

From the 1950s to the 1970s, the increase in the standard of living enabled most homes in Europe to possess the basic modern comforts: fridge, washing machine, dishwasher, television, car etc. Since the 1970s there has been no new significant addition to the list – unless we consider the micro-wave oven and the plastic salad shaker as major domestic revolutions. On the other hand these last two decades have been marked by an incredible informatics revolution, with the invasion of computers and the increasing number of television stations with satellites serving them. The massive reduction in industrial employment associated with this societal change has grow over the coming years. Our societies will have to humbly face the fact that they have been incapable of assuming the social consequences of the scientific and technical progress they engendered and continue to encourage. By going forward more and more quickly and refusing to think about the situation we have brought about we are creating unacceptable social situations, like the co-existence of 'yuppies' and the 'new poor' through flagrant imbalances in our society.

## *Ethics*

Our societies have not yet been able to come to grips with the ethical problems arising out of this technico-scientific revolution – people are no longer manually enslaved to a machine but intellectually enslaved to their computer; the threat to individual freedom; the difficulty of adapting to rapidly changing technologies and machines; the consequences of computer disorders and breakdowns; the capability of bugging and decoding the most sophisticated programmes; the dangers of destabilising the international markets (as happened on 'Black Monday' in October 1987). And television, which could have been a prodigious cultural vector, has become a way of selling food and nappies. With extremely sophisticated means it produces worse than mediocre programmes. And perhaps worst of all, it ignores two of the basic human needs – being part of nature and spiritual fulfilment.

We have not yet dared to analyse objectively and with humility the insidious consequences of our communication societies. There is an urgent need to set up – for communications and the media – committees on ethics such as those which already exist to study the problems posed by the evolution of human biology.

## *Humans and life*

If the end of the nineteenth century was typified by problems between the human and the natural, our era is marked by problems between humans and life, particularly their own life. Progress in biology and genetics mean that we can now produce babies how and when we like, male or female, *in vivo* or *in vitro*, with or without parents. Humans can be 'improved' just as cultivated plants have been in one of biology's great success stories.

But what will 'human improvement' be like? If birth can be manipulated, what about death? In short, we are now faced with problems we did not foresee and cannot control, especially when they are compounded by unpredictable factors like the insidious and cruel epidemic of AIDS.

To these and other questions relating to the meaning and future of science the scientific community is trying to find answers.

### *The emergence of a new spirituality*

The last two centuries have been marked by a constant process of secularisation. As the 21st century dawns, we are going to see a resurgence of the spiritual.

The nineteenth century claimed to have erased what had been part of human existence since time immemorial – the sacred and the spiritual dimension. Are these essential components of human beings? Certainly the proliferation of sects, and perhaps even the renaissance of Islamic fundamentalism, might be seen as a reaction against the deep and widespread materialism of societies with a high degree of scientific and technological progress and as a reaction against the institutions of these societies which, exclusively preoccupied with production and consumption, do not take other human facets into account – such as the spiritual – and only consider them as marginal and individual.

## Solidarity for the 21st century

The time has come to dispel a purely Darwinian and Manichean view of social structures. For what Darwin did not see was that nature survives not only through struggle, but through solidarity. As ecology progresses as a scientific discipline it is bringing this to light. The latest known example is the ability of trees to tell each other, through gas messages, of the arrival of a predator.

In the 21st century we shall need urgently to integrate solidarity into our social fabric at all levels: between citizens in a country; between countries in the same part of the world, and first in the European Community; between North and South. It is clear that the violence of economic competition between 'overdeveloped' regions, like the United States, Europe and Southeast Asia, will require armistices, negotiation and agreement if it is to be curbed and we are to survive.

Are the new religious ideologies taking the place of the dying political ones? It seems to me that we must not replace, but transcend such dialectical opposites. This would require working towards the emergence both of individual consciousness and a new collective consciousness. We would need to safeguard the traditional values of the State of Law and widen the scope for individual freedom. The old axioms of 'Others work for me – and good for me' and 'I work for me – and too bad for the others' would have to give way to a third: 'I work to transcend myself, to make myself little by little master of that which weighs me down and constrains me, so that I can create a productive dialogue with others, when the tyranny of "Me first" has been conquered in myself.' Such an approach, involving individual and collective consciousness, opens out naturally to the solidarity needed for the third millennium.

## *A few ingredients for a new world*

Our three basic needs, as the 21st century dawns, will be:

- Solidarity to build Europe and fight new forms of poverty, especially in the Third World;
- Ethical assessment of science and technology leading to their better use;
- Consideration of the spiritual dimension of humankind.

The ultimate aim in life, both individually and collectively, is not just economic and social progress, nor scientific and technical progress. It is above all a courageous and permanent self-questioning – that which, a few centuries ago, they called 'progress'. The success of this progress depends on each of us, and more precisely, on what is in the deepest recesses of our hearts. Pierre Emmanuel said: 'Changing your heart is changing your life'. If we bring about this change together, we will indeed change life.

So there is hope of a genuine spiritual revival, based on secular traditions and in the spirit of the first centuries of Christianity. Art will help, because it is free, and will continue its timeless role of revealing the most secret of trends and the profoundest of hopes of a society or an age.

As André Malraux said: 'There will not be a 21st century if it is not spiritual.'

Chapter 19

# Environmental protection: a labour of ethics

by Günter Altner

Ethics as the problem of what we may do and what we should achieve places a question mark after the actuality of what has been done and what is still developing. Moreover, ethics as the problem of what we should do challenges the self-evident and sets us thinking about new responsibilities and duties.

## Discovering nature's intrinsic value

Compared to the last two decades, today we are emerging from an exciting period of public reflection that has been triggered by our evolving ethical principles and related demands for substantive change in science, politics and society. A case in point is the ecological movement the call for recognition of the intrinsic value of nature and the need to protect it. It all began with the 'ecological imperative' first put in words by Hartmut Bossel in 1978: 'Act in such a way as to ensure that the claim to survival of all existing and future living systems is met.' After that there was no holding people back. Once the principle had been stated, the debate moved into increasingly intricate spheres while a call went out for a more ecological approach to technological development, production and politics – a call which has found its way into a wide range of specific programmes, incorporating some quite extreme positions.

For example, speaking at a jubilee congress of the Hoechst chemical company in Frankfurt am Main, philosopher Hans Jonas made an impassioned plea in favour of 'holy fear' as the proper attitude of modern people vis-à-vis the multiplicity of life: 'We must learn to fear and tremble again, and even if we reject God, fear the holy.' (Jonas, 1984). Jonas reminded his audience that we did not create things, that things were put at our disposal and so had a claim on us for protection.

In fact, Jonas was exhorting us to reverence for life much as Albert Schweitzer did earlier this century in words still remembered by many: 'I am Life, that wants to live, in the midst of Life, that also wants to live'. Schweitzer's commandment of reverence for life is based on the matter-of-fact recognition of the fact that life is always at the expense of other life. But, because life can be experienced as an elementary value in the sense of existence and preservation, the sorrow of competition for survival brings with it a duty to compensate and spare where we can.

'Peace with nature', a Kantian concept devised by Klaus Meyer-Abich (1984) also implies a duty-bound relationship between the human race and nature: 'Human beings, animals, plants and the elements are related in the history of nature and together they form a natural community in law. The intrinsic value of the natural environment is expressed in human laws.' Meyer-Abich takes the development of ethical consciousness one step further when he speaks of the need to devise appropriate legal frameworks and legislation to protect the intrinsic value of nature as discovered by humankind. Nature, assuming it has intrinsic value, cannot be regarded merely as the 'object' of legal duties, it must also enjoy the status of a legal 'subject' having original rights of its own which people acting as legal representatives can sue to protect.

Jürgen Dahl (1987/88) has no doubt best expressed the feelings of many concerned people today in pronouncing the agnostic's position: 'The agnostic, in his dealings with all that is "incomprehensible" in the world, with living creatures and genes, with the atomic structure of substance, with the forces and laws of matter, proceeds with the utmost caution.' In this scenario, the end product of 'ignorance' is not indifference, but care and concern for natural things.

Lastly, these exhortations to revere life are clearly compatible with the Christian view of the world as God's creation and the human race as its steward.

Generally speaking, then, we can say that the problem of human alienation from nature, as technological and industrial progress takes its toll, is now undergoing a critical debate on human responsibility for nature and an ethical reassessment. I believe that we should fear that which we have not made; that which, despite our techno-industrial posturing, must remain out of reach although it is the foundation of our existence. The classical, ethical relationship in the I-Thou society has become more polarised as a result of the recognition of nature as a claimant on humankind, and this has opened up new vistas and new options in areas such as energy, transport, alternative agricultural and chemical policies.

## The practical consequences of formulating alternative concepts – an attempt at a morphological approach

During the past ten years, the idea of alternative technology has nowhere been more to the forefront than in the field of energy. Traditional energy policy was geared to demand. It sought to stimulate economic growth through steadily rising primary energy demand and the building of gigantic new power plants. Boosting the development of nuclear energy was in keeping with this policy.

The appearance of the anti-nuclear lobby on the scene threw a policy alternative into the ring. Citizens and scientists alike stressed the advantages of an energy policy based on more efficient use of energy, decentralisation of the old supply structures and the gradual development of renewable energy sources. There is reliable evidence, not least from the German Federal Parliament's (Bundestag) energy experts, that economic growth is possible even if primary energy demand goes down. This is a vital prerequisite for qualitative growth in which we shall conserve finite resources and the environment while stimulating employment.

One of the salient features of an alternative approach to technological and economic development is the principle of fair cost, in which the indirect costs of different technological strategies (environmental burden, disruption of nature) are taken into account.

Similarly, transport policy is taking a new turn, questioning the justice of sacrificing the environment on the altar of mobility and speed. In concrete terms, the fight against motor vehicle exhaust and lead emissions, noise, and the invasion of the countryside by new motorways will mean transporting more goods by rail, improved public transport, more bicycle paths, etc.

Agricultural policy is also up for reform as nature reasserts her rights against exploitation. Artificially high prices for agricultural outputs have led to intensive farming with high chemical inputs which are resulting in acid soil, contaminated drinking water and the disappearance of many species of plant, animal and insect life. New, ecologically-oriented demands for agriculture include financial support for small and medium-sized family farms, abolition of farm surpluses by curbing the use of fertilisers and pesticides, and a stop to the further fragmentation of the countryside by urban development.

On the chemicals front, an alternative policy would be based on the awareness of ecological cycles and a metabolic balance with nature, which would increase life's chances of survival on the evolutionary plane. It will have to address such issues as quantitative risk assessment, toxicological and ecotoxicological risks, waste management and the development of a low-risk chemical industry.

Now that we have looked at the morphology of the ecological crossroads, it is time to see how ethics can be brought to bear on our prospects for the future.

## Ethics: methodological reflections on designing the future

Ethics, as the search for the right way to act, questions the past and projects into the future. Ethics dares to take seriously the apparently utopian precisely because human beings – no matter how much they may want to carry the past over into the future – are the actors, the seekers, the risk-takers, the 'open' element. All ethical systems, the religious and the secular, the conservative and the progressive, think alike on this. Each system of ethics refers to basic premises which cannot be verified. But each system also thrives on the gap between practices and fundamental hopes and duties – whether these concern justice, solidarity, love, peace or reverence for life. In its projections, each system mixes memory and hope, past and future in a dynamic whole.

Scientific rationality and prediction, on the other hand, only deal in the calculable past and the attainable future. That is not a very large section of the full spectrum of multidimensional time. This, the 'corridor' used by objective rationality is, in a sense, the extended present; that which is objective, unchangeable, reproduceable in spite of the bewildering march of time. In effect, it is the castration and reduction of multidimensional time to suit the premises of objective analysis. Thus, the dynamics of reality in the forcefield between past and future is argued away and consigned to the rubbish heap as unverifiably complex. For example, many people inappropriately define this nebulous area as the irrational, which must be rejected. Objective rationality does not include the past and still less the future to the extent required by ethical systems.

High time, then, that ethics should come to present a challenge to technical rationality. And the more future-oriented and utopian the ethical system, the more it allows itself to be guided by the possible which does not yet exist – for example peace – the greater will be the challenge to scientific and technical rationality and their 'small' opportunities. And since we are referring to hopes and opportunities raised by ethics, it is clear that however multifarious, ethics can never be merely arbitrary.

Building on a set of fundamental principles, ethics demand that we replace what has been achieved, or not been achieved, with what can become possible in the future. This can even go so far as to replace a fundamental principle: Albert Schweitzer replaced 'love thy neighbour' with 'reverence for life'. Since what has been done is the counterpart of what should be done, and since what should be done is a challenge to what has been done, an ethical system thus develops its own creative rationality. Progressive ethics are rooted in what should be done in the future, the hoped for, the utopian. It would be quite ridiculous, therefore, to try to set the principle of responsibility against the principle of hope.

Since we are confronted by the fact that, today, the traditional duties of human and social tolerance are coupled with new goals in the shape of international, generative and ecological tolerance, ethical assessment has become even more complicated. We are dealing here with real, conflicting goals which will have to be carefully researched, although we may be fantasising about a state of peace in which humans and nature walk hand in hand and, in biblical terms, our grandchildren can play safely at the entrance to the snake pit and swords be beaten into ploughshares. Hans Jonas has rightly pointed out that the ethical malevolence of techno-industrial progress resides precisely in the fact that innocent-looking ploughshares can cause untold damage, just as 'safe' propellant gases can tear apart the earth's protective ozone layer.

When we search the future to assess consequences and tolerances, we should do well to seek out the plane of stress between the hidden and the visible; between the human race and nature, between the present and an imaginable future; between our closed, consumer structures and open co-operative systems; between the detailed empirical approach and holistic ecology; and also the stress between the knowledge that life is the highest good and yet to death must seem a canker. If we can but place ourselves in the middle of this plane of stress, we will see the future as a promised land, a land on whose border we stand but which still lies far away.

Such an utopian ethical system must be based on multiplicity and public participation. It must lend an ear to those who stand up for dumb nature and plead for ecological and social protection, and to those who would extend our consumer and interest group oriented society and so lock the past onto the future.

## Ethics as an open process of weighing pros and cons

In recent years, Reinhard Überhorst (1986) has repeatedly stressed the need for a discursive style of politics in respect of scientific and technological progress. He distinquishes between 'positional' politics and 'discursive' politics. According to Überhorst, persons holding 'positional' political views know what they want and demand a consistent policy line. Discursive politics, on the other hand, offers a system which listens to and accommodates open questions and alternative courses of action. Positional politics either does not tolerate objections or puts objectors in the position of opponents. Discursive politics looks at objections, takes them in its stride, and is willing to include objectors as potential partners and participants in the decision-making process. Positional politics seeks immunity from alternatives, discursive politics seeks to accommodate alternatives.

As long as people in the ecological movement and their alternative ways of looking at technological and environmental policy-making are not given their rightful place in the decision-making process, discursive politics is lamed by the lack of an ecological perspective. Ecologically oriented politics is democratic, participatory politics. It is politics which will hear the defence of the dumb environment even though the defenders are in a minority. Politics as practised by the special interest lobbies is not consistent with democratic procedures, unless we believe that our dawning respect for life is stuff and nonsense.

Industrial lobbies and public authorities are trying hard to adapt their political style to a more ecology-conscious public. But we all know that the vital alternatives on which to base preventive environmental policies were never hatched in Parliament, universities or industry. What we need is a new policy style which overtly thinks in terms of alternatives and weighs the pros and cons of different solutions. If we take this seriously, then we shall increase the transparency of democratic decision-making and reduce the element of compulsion. This means, of course, that we make full use of civil rights, but equally we must think about new participatory models of government which can contribute to even more openness and democracy in an ecological policy.

Some steps might be taken to assist this development. First, there must be greater use of public inquiry bodies, including a parliamentary group on the lines of the U.S. Congress Office of Technology Assessment. These bodies must incorporate strong alternative, ecological and social interests.

Second, there should be more public and more democratic licensing procedures for major projects with potential environmental impacts, and the possibility of declaring moratoria, research and production stops. We need, to quote Hans Jonas, a 'stay of execution a few steps in advance of progress'.

A prerequisite for the establishment of appropriate value standards for progress without exploitation depends on our ability to give ourselves and Nature time – her time, our ability to hold on and grab our chance of a different relationship. Our attempt to conquer Nature's time with the help of our calculating wits and to escape the laws of time in our own existence has, as the current crisis of human survival clearly shows, failed dismally. Ecology, as an expression of giving ourselves time, of moving together with nature towards the future, is possible only if we become ethically aware that existence, in the long run, must be a matter of receiving, not disposing. The recognition that nature cannot meet our every wish can help us cope with and overcome the manipulative genius of scientific and technological planning.

## References


Bossel, H., *Bürgerinitiativen entwerfen die Zukunft – Neue Leitbilder, neue Werte,* 30 Szenarien, Frankfurt am Main, 1978, p. 181.

Dahl, J., in *Scheidewege,* vol. 17, 1987/88, pp. 58–9.

Jonas, H., in *International Symposium of the Hoechst Corporation: Am Beginn des 2. Jahrhundert - Hoechst-Pharma,* 1984, p. 25.

Meyer-Abich, Kl. M., *Wege zum Frieden mit der Natur. Praktische Naturphilosophie für die Umweltpolitik,* Munich, 1984, pp. 190–91.

Überhorst, R., 'Technologiepolitik – Was wäre das? Über Dissens und Meinungsstreit als Noch-nicht-Instrumente der sozialen Kontrolle der Gentechnik', in Kollek, R., Tappeser, B., Altner, G. (eds), *Die ungeklärten Gefahrenpotentiale der Gentechnologie,* Munich, 1986, p. 202 ff.

Chapter 20

# Scientific commitment and the crisis in the environment

by Federico Mayor

> One fact, more than any other, which should not be overlooked is that if man, as a thinking, contemplative being, were banished from the surface of the earth, then the sublime and moving spectacle of nature would be nothing more than a sad and silent scene ... the universe would be mute, enfolded in silence and night. All would be transformed into a vast and lonely wilderness where dim and muffled events would remain unobserved ... .

The message of hope bequeathed by Diderot and other great men of the eighteenth century – the Enlightenment – was of a rational harmony between man and nature. What has happened in the last two hundred years that today, having conquered the moon and the depths of the oceans, we look around, anxious, wondering if we have not failed in the challenge we inherited? Never before in human history have there been in so short a time so many upheavals, irreversible changes and radical transformations as we have seen in the past quarter of a century. Social revolutions have wiped out old orders, industrial revolutions have transformed means of production, and there has been a dizzy acceleration in scientific and technological progress, whose benefits have gone hand in hand with devastating effects on people and the environment. It is almost as if human beings, casting off the shoes in which they had advanced, step by step, through the ages, had suddenly put on their seven–league boots and made giant strides.

With these upheavals has come a new perception of our world. No longer do we see geographical areas and their resources as huge, almost infinite reservoirs on which society can draw at will for its own development.

### *The birth of ecology*

The German scholar Ernst Haeckel coined the word 'ecology' in 1869 to denote the study of relationships between a given organism and its environment. Until then, scientists from many disciplines had painstakingly and systematically classified natural resources and their properties, but the dynamic relationships between the different components of the living world – including that between human beings and the earth, their life support – had not been comprehensively studied.

Most scientific disciplines are like trees, with branches growing out of a main trunk and twigs sprouting out of the branches. Ecology is different. We need to look at it as a number of roots – botany, zoology, earth sciences, physical geography, microbiology, then human geography, sociology, psychology and economics – converging into one trunk. So the ecological trunk is not as coherent or homogeneous as that of the other sciences, since the disciplines which make it up have not yet merged into a single integrated approach. But these converging roots make it particularly flexible and effective in dealing with the increasingly complex problems of the environment, where action on one element can trigger off a chain reaction.

As the discipline of ecology has developed over the last 50 years so the concept of environment has clearly taken shape as the general natural, physical and social context of human life and action, including, but no longer limited to, natural resources. Thus, those very sciences that were the taproots of ecology have developed into the environmental sciences.

## A world in imbalance

While human society is now organised globally, it is riddled with major disparities from one region to another, and particularly between developed and developing countries. This form of organisation rests on a technological system which increases its efficiency at both the national and the international levels, by introducing economic competition among its agents. Each of them seeks to take maximum advantage of what technology has to offer, while at the same time keeping costs as low as possible, notably by letting others bear as many of these costs as possible. The results of this are widespread competition and growing imbalances between societies themselves and between societies and nature.

This results in uncertainty and anxiety about the future, expressed by some as a 'great fear of the year 2000'. Is this only because of the deterioration of the physical and biological environment? I am not sure. I think that what we call the environmental crisis is only one aspect – a major one admittedly – of a more general crisis of civilisation.

Faced with a changing world, with shifting horizons and deep social and economic inequalities, where the excesses of some provide a day-to-day contrast with the poverty of so many others, people are beginning to perceive differently their destiny and the space in which it unfolds and to wonder about the direction history is taking, about spiritual goals and material development.

Times of crisis, more than others, are rich in positive potential, and I firmly believe this potential can be realised. But the formula is neither simple nor obvious. We have to see the crux of the crisis we are going through – both societal and economic – as the interface between people, their environment and their desire not only to develop their economy but also to improve the quality of their lives. Only then can we hope to begin to draw up a common, pragmatic plan of action to resolve the crisis.

## The Brundtland Report

New concepts and new instruments are being defined to bring about effective joint action, involving collaboration between developed and developing countries. In this respect the report of the United Nations World Commission on Environment and Development (better known as the 'Brundtland Report', after the Chairwoman of the Commission, Mrs Gro Harlem Brundtland, Prime Minister of Norway) is of great importance.

An idea from this report which seems to me to be of prime importance is the possibility for developing countries to maintain their economic and social development while ensuring the long-term conservation of the basic natural resources on which their development depends. This is the idea of sustainable development, which may be seen as a 'concerted effort to meet present needs without jeopardising future needs' and, more broadly, as a framework for the integration of environment policies and development strategies.

When we speak of development, we often think only of the economic growth of the third world on present-day foundations. Yet the concept of sustainable development presupposes major changes in the policies pursued by all countries – both rich and poor. It would not mean an end to economic growth – far from it – but rather ensuring that this growth no longer wastes resources and threatens the environment. If economic progress at last has due regard for its ecological roots, then the defence of the environment will be structurally linked to sustainable development.

I am not suggesting either that an ideal development model is being put forward, because social systems, economic conditions and ecological realities vary from country to country and each country has to find its own path. Yet no country can develop in isolation. In the long term, international relations will have to change radically to allow a more balanced, equitable exchange and flow of goods, capital and technology while at the same time taking greater account of environmental necessities.

The Brundtland Report states that sustainable development requires the introduction of an economic system capable of generating surpluses and permanently creating technical skills, a social system capable of reducing the tensions created by the imbalances in present growth, a production system that respects the obligation to preserve the ecological base of economic growth, an international system fostering equitable patterns of trade and finance, and a flexible administrative system capable of self-correction.

These recommendations are preceded by a definition of sustainable development which aims to 'promote harmony among human beings and between humanity and nature'. We are reminded of Diderot's words.

Thus the Brundtland Report reflects the highly ethical concerns of its writers and their profound trust in the virtues of reason. While the practical means needed to carry out such a complex task are not immediately apparent, we are nevertheless now under the obligation to identify them. And by 'we' I mean not only our collective responsibilities in whatever social role we play, but also our duties as individuals.

## The role of the scientist

Politicians, scientists and intellectuals have social roles and a moral status which go beyond their role as individuals. Their ideas and actions may influence major currents of opinion, even whole populations. Their responsibilities are therefore wider and more binding than those of the ordinary run of people.

Science today is no longer a body of knowledge, a method of discovery reserved for an élite. It is a socio-cultural phenomenon of vast proportions which is increasingly in evidence in all aspects of life in today's societies. As such, it is beginning to create problems and generate contradictions. Science has such a major impact on modern society not merely because of the image of reality it projects, but above all because it has engendered technology, that aggregate of equipment and practices in which our existences have become enmeshed and which determine directly our lifestyles and indirectly our perceptions and value systems. The development of science and technology has shaken the very foundations of cultures by introducing new knowledge and new practices.

We therefore need to consider simultaneously the socio-economic, political and technological structures, if we are to keep the world viable for ourselves and future generations. This is a political task, with science as the main means of action. But the events which have marked the history of science and technology are vastly different from those which most deeply characterise a culture, and the former can have a highly destructuring effect on the latter. This is the danger awaiting many cultures whose identities we must protect – just as we protect endangered species of plants or animals – in order to ensure present and future ecological balance.

How then do science, technology and cultures interact, and how will cultures be affected by this interaction? Will their specific identities gradually disintegrate, or will there be a radical reorganisation of their ethical and aesthetic components? These are questions which concern me particularly because the outcome of processes at work today, one way or the other, will affect not only present but future generations. It is here that the moral responsibility of intellectuals in general and scientists in particular comes into play, for it is their thinking and action which will decide which of the various possibilities will be followed up.

The scientific community must thus act quickly, because the effects of irrationality, competition and egotism are already becoming apparent in imbalances which are mortgaging the future of several generations. They have a duty to alert public opinion and governments to problems facing humanity, and to provide the most reliable and unimpeachable scientific basis for international standard setting action. Scientists are not starting from scratch. Action has already been taken: scientific programmes have been in progresss – some for twenty years now – and efforts have been made to acquire more knowledge about land and marine resources and hence to manage them better.

A good recent example was when scientists noted a depletion in the ozone layer and concluded that the increasing use of chlorofluorocarbons (CFCs), especialy in aerosols, could have contributed to it. They felt that the probability was sufficiently strong to warrant a joint effort on their part to convince governments to undertake to reduce the production of CFCs, despite the possible economic consequences of such a limitation.

But much remains to be done concerning, for example, the role and production of carbon dioxide and its impact on energy production, the transport of crude oil and the volume of waste accumulating on the sea beds, the blanket use of pesticides and herbicides, forest die-back and acid rain. Standard-setting activities, however, can only be carried through by nations, which at times find it difficult to do so because of the high cost of implemention. Hence the absolute necessity for a scientific basis for legislation. States will be all the more inclined to meet their obligations if supported by research that reveals the contribution these activities can make to better management of the environment and natural resources.

## *The contribution of Unesco to environmental protection*

Unesco was established as a specialised agency within the United Nations system to promote peace by fostering dialogue and mutual understanding among peoples through education, science and culture. One of Unesco's three core mandates is therefore science, and it is through the role of scientific research as a source of knowledge and a basis for the rational management of resources that the organisation's contribution to environmental protection should be seen, in close co-operation with the United Nations Environment Programme (UNEP) which was set up to stimulate and co-ordinate programmes on the environment throughout the United Nations.

Within this framework, Unesco is at present carrying out four intergovernmental scientific programmes on environment and natural resources:

- the International Geological Correlation Programme, conducted jointly with the International Union of Geological Sciences, which aims to analyse phenomena in the earth's crust that have a direct bearing on the distribution of mineral and fuel resources;
- the International Hydrological Programme, which seeks to identify the basis for the rational long-term management of water resources;
- the Intergovernmental Oceanographic Commission, aimed at better defining the mechanisms which govern the oceans and their resources, as well as their effects on climate;
- the Intergovernmental Programme on Man and the Biosphere, an interdisciplinary ecological programme of research, training and demonstration which seeks, through pilot projects, comparative studies and the setting up of biosphere reserves, to provide practical methods for sustainable development through the rational management of terrestrial and aquatic ecosystems.

These programmes share a certain number of features which need to be stressed. They all enjoy the active involvement of both developed and developing countries. They are designed by intergovernmental scientific bodies, but are carried out by the countries themselves, usually through national committees made up of the appropriate governmental department, universities and research institutes. They develop multilateral co-operation through permanent secretariats in Unesco itself, but encourage bilateral co-operation between one national committee and another – both between

North and South and between different developing countries. They are problem-oriented research programmes with an interdisciplinary approach, and therefore encourage constant interaction between researchers on the one hand and planners and decision-makers on the other, thus facilitating the effective use of research findings. Finally they provide opportunities for interinstitutional co-operation with and between relevant UN bodies, non-governmental scientific organisations and the populations of the countries involved.

## The challenge facing us

There is, then, a growing international awareness of the global threats to our environment and of the actions needed to counter them.

The challenges facing us remain enormous, however, and we have to make a much greater effort, not only because of the dangers that are clearly emerging, but also because the action they make necessary comes up against tremendous obstacles stemming from human nature, societal pressures and the mechanisms of economic competition. Such action conflicts with habits and inertia because it entails major changes in our behaviour, production and consumption. It also runs counter, in certain cases, to economic interests which take advantage of the pressure of international competition to override ecological considerations. None of these obstacles must stop us. Our responsibility is global, both in space and time. It is at once international and intergenerational. We cannot shirk it.

I appeal finally to all scientists, researchers and teachers. Speak out! Add to the moral imperative the authority of science; awaken people's minds and alert their consciences to what is at stake in our common future. Call forth the intelligence that is in us all, so as to overcome egotism, defeat inertia and work for the development of our societies.

# Part III

# Politics and Politicians

Chapter 21

# Radioactivity with regard to the production and use of nuclear weapons: its impact on health

by Emile Tockert

On 6 August 1945 a nuclear weapon was used for the first time against humanity. A thirteen kiloton $uranium^{235}$ fission bomb exploded in the sky over Hiroshima. Three days later, a 22 kiloton $plutonium^{239}$ bomb was dropped on Nagasaki. The civil population of Hiroshima in the area covered by the first blast was about 300,000, of which 68,000 were killed and 76,000 injured immediately. The number of deaths had risen to 140,000 by the end of 1945 and 200,000 at the end of 1950. It was only later that cancers began to appear.

## The specificity of nuclear weapons

The energy liberated during a nuclear explosion is of three types; fifty per cent in a shock wave which causes most physical damage, thirty-five per cent in heat which causes burns and fires, fifteen per cent in radioactive radiation – the specificity of nuclear bombs. While the shock and heat waves are responsible for immediate deaths and injuries, radioactivity is the cause of acute and early radiation sickness and also delayed abnormalities in the years, or even decades, after exposure.

Radioactive radiation gets to people in two ways. First, during the explosion intense radiation is emitted with a very high penetrating power. After this the radioactive particles, scattered in the atmosphere, fall to earth. Through the food chain this radiation accumulates in the human organism and irradiates the body from the inside. The global consequences on the human organism of these different effects of an explosion are increased by their synergy.

### *How does radioactivity act on our organism*

Unstable isotopes used in nuclear fission or fusion are transformed and give off energy in the form of radiation – notably $\alpha$ and $\beta$ particles, $\gamma$ rays and neutrons.

The $\alpha$ and $\beta$ particles do not have great penetrating power, but they enter our organism through inhalation or ingestion, and once there, fixed and concentrated, they can damage cells with which they come into contact. Both $\gamma$ rays and neutrons have great penetrating power and through ionisation modify the atomic structure of cell molecules.

Cells are the most radiosensitive in their multiplication phase. In mitosis, chromosomes in the process of reproduction are particularly at risk, and this explains, in part, why organs which have permanent cellular renewal can be damaged more than others. In the digestive tract the top layer of the mucous membranes renews itself continuously. In bone marrow, stem cells multiply constantly to produce different blood lines.

This mechanism explains both delayed and transmissible (i.e. hereditary) abnormalities. The function of the cell is programmed by the genetic code written into the chromosomes, and if this code is disrupted, the cell no longer recognises its function, becomes disturbed and may be radically altered over the years, i.e. become cancerous. If it is a reproductive or embryonic cell, the disrupted code can be transmitted to the daughter cells all the way down the line, resulting in possible congenital and/or hereditary abnormalities. Also, the cells in our central nervous system are very sensitive to the action of ionising radiation.

Depending on the amount of exposure, there are three types of acute radiation sickness.

- *Neurological:* massive irradiation of 5,000 rads[1] or more causes convulsions, coma and death in a few hours; with between 4,500 and 1,500 rads, sickness develops in a less acute form: lethargy, then coma, then death in a few days.
- *Intestinal:* one week after a dose of 400 to 500 rads, serious digestive problems appear. Following the destruction of the epithelium in the intestine, profuse and bleeding diarrhoea occurs causing serious, even

---

1 A rad is a unit of dose – the energy absorbed per unit mass. 1 rad = 0.01 GY. The LD 50 (i.e. where fifty per cent of an exposed adult population would die) is 450 rads.

lethal, dehydration. The risks of septicemia are high because of the destruction of the mucous barrier separating the intestine from the rest of the organism.

- *Medullary:* bone marrow generates blood cells, and a dose of more than 150 rads destroys it in varying degrees. After a ten-day latency period, reduced and non-regenerated blood cells are incapable of fulfilling their physiological functions. An insufficiency in blood platelets causes external and internal bleeding. White corpuscles, the carriers of immunity, can no longer defend the organism against infection. If this immune deficiency affects whole populations whose organisation and medical infrastructure has collapsed, there will be epidemics.

Delayed abnormalities from radioactive radiation are typified by problems of embryogenesis and cancer. The embryo and the foetus can be damaged both by direct irradiation and by irradiation from the mother's body which has absorbed radioactive substances. Most pregnant Japanese women who were irradiated with more than 200 rads before the fifteenth week of pregnancy gave birth to children with malformations – particularly related to brain development. Among the survivors, forty-four per cent had microcephaly accompanied by mental deficiencies. In more advanced pregnancies, neo-natal and infantile mortality were abnormally high (Wood, 1967; Kato, 1969).

The number of leukaemias was statistically higher than average and reached a peak six years after the two nuclear explosions. The latency period of solid tumours was longer, and it was only twenty to twenty-five years later that an unusually high rate of cancers was noted, particularly of the lungs, thyroid and bones. The epidemiological study of the cancerous illnesses observed after Hiroshima enables us to establish a clear link between the assumed dose of exposure and the total number of cancers.

However, to this day, there has been no proven evidence of a significant increase in genetic damage. Experimental irradiation of animals and human cell cultures causes a mutation rate proportional to the dose used. The absence of excessive genetic damage in the descendants of the survivors of Hiroshima may be explained by a number of factors. Most of the victims exposed to strong doses died in the firestorm which lasted six hours. Some of the survivors became sterile. Transmissible abnormalities, mostly recessive, tend to appear after several generations.

## The dangers of nuclear testing

The development and improvement of nuclear weapons through the testing they require have direct consequences on our environment and health.

Between 1945 and April 1986, the five nuclear powers carried out 1,618 nuclear tests – USA: 804, USSR: 604, UK: 39, France: 142, China: 30, and India: 1. Until 1963, when the Limited Test Ban Treaty was concluded, the two superpowers carried out their tests in the atmosphere. The Treaty banned tests in the atmosphere but not underground. France halted its tests in the atmosphere in 1976 and China in 1981.

From the 1950s on, scientists tried to draw attention to the dangers of radioactive fallout. Professor Linus Pauling, having collected the signatures of more than 9,000 eminent scientists, led a decisive campaign. The Physicians for Social Responsibility (PSR), out of which the future IPPNW was to grow, collected and analyzed several thousand milk teeth in St. Louis (USA), located in a fallout area. The presence of strontium$^{90}$ was established. This radioactive substance behaves like calcium in that it moves up the food chain through milk and becomes fixed in the organism of the child in teeth and bones.

Such campaigns, supplemented with the publication of medical papers on the subject, helped to bring about President Kennedy's unilateral decision, on 10 June 1963, to call a halt to tests in the atmosphere. Three weeks later, the Soviet Union did the same.

Since then, underground testing has gone on at the rate of about 30 to 50 explosions per year until 1986. But it would be unwise to think that underground tests hold no danger, for they can also give rise to radioactive discharges into the atmosphere. There were ninty-seven such 'ventings' between 1964 and 1970, of which thirty-one were beyond the perimeter of the test site. On two occasions, the fallout reached Canada.

To what extent does radioactive fallout from tests have consequences on human health? It is difficult to show a direct correlation between such fallout and the onset of radiation-induced illness for numerous reasons:

(1) It is impossible to prove that a given case of cancer is the specific result of radioactive pollution.
(2) The latency period makes etiological research difficult.
(3) Cancer is in constant progression as a result, amongst other things, of a variety of nuisances, of our eating habits and of increased longevity.

However, many studies have been made, and are still being made, of the effects of nuclear testing on health. What follows is a sample of representative studies carried out around two testing sites.

## *Nevada and Bikini: the effects go on*

Starting in 1951, more than 180 tests were carried out in Nevada. At least 87 led to radioactive contamination outside the test site – notably the south-west of the State of Utah where several studies subsequently noted an increase in cases of leukaemia. One study revealed twenty-eight cases between 1951 and 1964 as against an expected nineteen. Another noted that the frequency of leukaemia deaths in children between 1951 and 1956 was 2.44 times higher than in the average population. But of particular interest was a study carried out among Mormons (Johnson, 1984) where, under normal circumstances, there are twenty-three per cent fewer cancers than in the general population – possibly due to the strict rules of the religion, and in particular abstinence from alcohol and tobacco.

After tests, and during the passage of radioactive clouds over the region, people living out of doors had already complained of burns to the eyes and skin and of sickness accompanied by vomiting. The study itself was made on a population of 4,125 Mormons between 1959 and 1980. 288 cases of cancer were reported as against an expected 179 – an overall increase of sixty-one per cent – and the growth rate with time tends to indicate that the peak, particularly for leukaemia, has not yet been reached. Most of these cases have been leukaemia, but amongst the solid cancers, the most frequent are lymphomas, melanomas and cancers of the thyroid.

In the late 1950s, nearly 250,000 American soldiers and about 150,000 civilians had 'front row seats' for different tests. An abnormally high rate of cancer has been noted among these people. On 10 May 1984 a Utah judge held that the United States Government had knowingly withheld the dangers of this voluntary exposure. It was sentenced to pay damages to nine cancer victims.

On 1 March 1954 the first test of a thermo-nuclear bomb was held – the Bravo test – when an H-bomb exploded on the ground in the Bikini atoll. A change in wind direction blew the radioactive cloud in the direction of the Marshall Islands, including Rongelap, where the inhabitants had been neither evacuated nor even warned, even though the wind change had been detected in time (Defence Nuclear Agency, 1954). Radioactive contamination was enormous, both in extent and in intensity – an area of 20,000 $km^2$ was exposed to a lethal dose of radiation. A few hours after the explosion, the ground in Rongelap was covered in a layer of ashes two to five centimetres deep, and the inhabitants of the island thought it was snow. Forty-eight hours later the inhabitants were evacuated, but already the first signs of radiation sickness had appeared: ninety per cent of the people had skin burns and most were suffering from diarrhoea and vomiting.

During the first few years after the explosion, the number of abortions and stillbirths doubled. Nine years later the first thyroid tumours appeared, affecting thirty-four per cent of the total population and seventy-seven per cent of the children. The land and the sea – from which the indigenous population takes its food – was severely polluted. The plankton was 58,000 times more radioactive than the seawater in one place studied.

The author of one study wrote in 1958: 'The habitation of these people on the island will afford most valuable ecological radiation data on human beings.' (Conard et al., 1957; Johnson, 1980).

## *Soviet and French testing: silence*

We do not have information about the health consequences of Soviet nuclear testing. Officially there have been no 'technical problems', but radiobiology and radioecology obey the same laws and pose the same problems everywhere.

The French authorities have been more than discreet about health and pollution hazards associated with their nuclear testing in the Pacific. The Mururoa atoll – called by some 'French Gruyère' – has been undermined by countless shock waves. It has been estimated that the atoll sinks two centimetres every year. In 1979 a 140 kiloton explosion started an earth tremor of 6.3 on the Richter scale, and caused a tidal wave in which seven people were killed or injured. In 1980 and 1981 plutonium escaped into the atmosphere when storms ripped away large areas of asphalt. As the atoll is full of plutonium waste, its disintegration would provoke massive radioactive pollution of the ocean.

All types of cancer are on the increase in the South Pacific, but as France refuses to cooperate with the South Pacific Conference and to pass on epidemiological data to the World Health Organization we can only base our information on what we learn from local people and hospitals.

## *Nuclear accidents*

The history of the military nuclear industry has been punctuated with accidents involving radioactive pollution. One striking incident took place on 21 January 1968 when a B-52 bomber, with four thermo-nuclear bombs on board, crashed on an ice floe in Thulé, Greenland. The auto-destruct mechanism brought about the release of at least twenty kilograms of plutonium. Eight hundred Danish and Eskimo workers removed the debris of the plane, and 600 containers holding 57 million litres of water and 277 containers with the debris of the plane were sent back to the United States. Official declarations assured the workers that there was 'no danger to man or animal and plant life'. But in December 1986 the Danish Prime Minister, Påul Schluter, ordered a study of the workers involved in the clearing-up operation. Five hundred are ill, with neurological, ocular, skin and respiratory problems, or a worsening of their general health. Ninety-eight of them have cancer (Bastian, 1986; Feldman, 1986).

All the examples I have given about testing and accidents are representative and are based on epidemiological studies. The overall picture suggests that many of the effects described will continue to be an integral part of conditions of life in the future and of the heritage we leave our children. It is also clear from these studies that in the vast majority of cases, the authorities have either minimised or even denied the dangers posed by the liberation of radioactive substances.

## International Physicians for the Prevention of Nuclear War

In 1962 a team of American doctors, including Professor Bernard Lown, the future co-founder of IPPNW, published an article in the New England Journal of Medicine on the medical consequences of a nuclear attack on a major city. Many other publications have followed, including, notably, the 1983 World Health Organization document 'Effects of nuclear war on health and health services'.

The conclusions of these analyses, based on medical criteria, were unanimous and irrefutable: in the event of a nuclear conflict, there can be no efficient medical aid. So as to remain faithful to our professional and deontological commitment, there is only one position open to us as doctors: to mobilise all our knowledge and influence to *prevent* this 'last epidemic' of humanity. It is this major challenge to the world medical community which the 180,000 doctors of IPPNW have taken up in almost 60 countries.

'Our aim is to alert physicians world-wide of the mortal peril to the public health. Our hope is that physicians will help educate their communities, for only an aroused and informed citizenry can change the course of events.' (B. Lown)

Since the beginning of our campaign, we have thought that the frantic arms race brings with it even now direct and indirect effects on human health. One of these is that nuclear dissuasion – which really means constant global nuclear threat – has serious negative psychological repercussions, particularly amongst young people.

The development of more and more sophisticated and powerful weapons requires increased military spending. In 1987, US$ 930 billion was invested in armaments. More than seventy per cent of all research carried out is military. The United Nations repeats endlessly that humanity cannot go on with the arms race and create proper living conditions for people at the same time. It is worthwhile remembering that the cost of the campaign to eliminate smallpox – one of the greatest scourges of our history – was about the same as one hour of global military spending. Because of the funds it diverts, the arms race can now be considered an undeclared war against the poor.

Finally I would like to recall the IPPNW position on nuclear testing.

Tests have an effect on our health. They are also a preparation for war. The United States needs to carry out less than one test per year to verify the state of its missiles, and two tests to study the effects of explosions (Joeck and York). Ten to fifteen per year are needed to develop new nuclear weapons systems. The same proportions would apply to the nuclear military programmes of other countries. It is clear then that testing is an essential condition to the building up of nuclear devices and important driving force within the nuclear arms race.

This is why IPPNW demands that all nuclear explosions be banned. Such a ban is verifiable by modern seismological techniques and hence would require no assumption of mutual trust. It would also put the safety of no country in jeopardy. It would be the first essential step – not only towards a halt to the arms race, but to a reversal of it.

## References


Bastian, T., *Atomkatastrophen und ihre Folgen,* Jungjohann-Verlag, 1986.

Baumann, R., 'Ökologische und medizinische Folgen der amerikanischen Atomtests auf dem Versuchsgelände in Nevada, Rundbrief *Ärzte Warnen vor dem Atomkrieg,* no. 19, Berlin.

Caldwell, G.G., et al., 'Leukaemia among participants in military manoeuvres at a nuclear bomb test – a preliminary report', *JAMA,* vol. 244, no. 14, 3 Oct. 1980.

Christoffel, J.D. and Swartzmann, J.D., 'Nuclear weapons testing fallout: proving causation for exposure injury', *Amer. Journal of Public Health,* vol. 76, no. 3, March 1986.

Conard, R.A., et al., 'Medical survey of Rongelap and Utirik people three years after exposure to radioactive fallout', Brookhaven National Laboratory, vol. 501, p. 22, Upton (NY), June 1958.

Ehrlich, P.R., Harte, J., Harwell, M.A., et al., 'Longterm biological consequences of nuclear war', *Science,* 2 vol. 22, 1983, pp. 1293–300,

Escalona, S.K., 'Children's responses to the nuclear war threat', *Children,* 1963, pp. 137–42.

Glasstone, S. and Dolan P., *The effects of atomic weapons,* U.S. Department of Defense and U.S. Energy Research and Development Administration, Washington, D.C., 1977.

Hiroo, Kato, 'Mortality in children exposed to the A-bombs while *in utero,* 1945–1969', *Amer. Journal of Epidemiology,* vol. 93, no. 6.

IPPNW, Proceedings of the first IPPNW congress, Virginia, (USA), 20 March 1981.

IPPNW, 'Nuclear testing at Mururoa', *Nuclear Issues*, no. 2, IPPNW.

IPPNW, *Impact of the threat of nuclear war on children and adolescents*, Proceedings of an International Research Symposium, IPPNW, 1984.

Ishimaru, T., et al., 'Dose-response relationship of neutrons and gamma-rays to leukaemia among atomic bomb survivors in Hiroshima and Nagasaki by type of leukaemia 1950–1971', *Radiation Research*, 1979, 77, pp. 377–94.

Joeck, N. and York, H.F., *Countdown on the comprehensive test ban*, University of California Press.

Johnson, C.J., 'Cancer incidence in an area of radioactive fallout downwind from the Nevada test site', *JAMA*, vol. 251, no. 2, 13 Jan. 1984.

Johnson, G., 'Paradise Lost', *Bulletin of the Atomic Scientists*, vol. 36, no. 10, 1980, p. 24.

Leaf, A., 'New perspectives on the medical consequences of nuclear war', *The New England Journal of Medicine*, vol. 315, no. 14, 1986, pp. 905–12.

Legget J.K., 'Geoscience and the feasibility of cheating on nuclear test ban treaties', *Modern Geology*, vol. 9, no. 4, 1985.

Liebow, et al., 'Pathology of the atomic bomb casualties', *Amer. Journal of Pathology*, 25, 1949, pp. 853–60.

Lyon, J.L., et al., 'Childhood leukaemias associated with fallout from nuclear testing', *The New England Journal of Medicine*, vol. 300, no. 8.

Resibois, A. and Joffroy, A., *Armes nucléaires: les médecins désarmés*, AMPGN (IPPNW), 1982.

Rotblat, J., 'Acute radiation mortality in a nuclear war', Institute of *Medicine: The medical implications of nuclear war*, National Academy Press, Washington, D.C., 1986, pp. 233–50.

Schwebel, M., 'Effects of the nuclear war threat on children and teenagers: implications for professionals', *Amer. J. Orthopsychiatry*, 1982, 52, pp. 608–18.

Sidel, V.W., 'Destruction before detonation: the impact of the arms race on health and health care', *The Lancet*, 7 Dec. 1985.

Sidel, V.W., Geiger, H.J. and Lown B., 'The physician's role in the postattack period', *New England Journal of Medicine*, vol. 266, 1962, pp. 1137–45.

Sivard, R.L., *World military and social expenditures 1987*, World Priorities.

Sykes, L. and Evernden, J., 'The verification of a comprehensive nuclear test ban', *Scientific American*, vol. 247, no. 4, pp. 29–37.

Turco, R.P., Toon, O.B., Ackerman, T.P., Pollack J.B. and Sagan, C., 'Nuclear winter: global consequences of multiple nuclear explosions, *Science*, vol. 222, 1983, pp. 1283–92.

Watanabe, S., 'Cancer and Leukaemia Developing Among Bomb Survivors', *Handbuch der allgemeiner Pathologie*, vol. 6, part 5, Springer-Verlag, Berlin, 1974.

Wood, J.W., Johnson K.G. and Yoskiaki, Omori., '*In utero* exposure to the Hiroshima atomic bomb', *Pediatrics*, vol. 39, March 1967.

World Health Organization, 'Effects of Nuclear war on health and health services: report of the International Committee of Experts in Medical Sciences and Public Health to implement resolution WHA.34.38.', WHO, Geneva, 1984.

Chapter 22

# Understanding our concept of nature

by Huguette Bouchardeau

Certain misunderstandings between technicians, decision-makers and leaders would disappear if we had a clearer and more rational idea of what 'nature' is. The confusion arises because throughout our history, from the Greeks and Romans onwards, the word has had two meanings.

## Mother Nature

The first is the concept of Mother Nature – a vast harmonious organism made up of everything that lives. A nature in harmony, taking us in, feeding us, but of which we human beings are only a small part. So when we talk of not attacking nature because it will get angry and react, or that we must obey nature's laws, or when we say we must have respect for all that lives – it is this concept of nature we are evoking.

Don't play with nature, we say, because we don't know what will happen if we destroy the balance that exists there. But this leads to our not doing anything at all to 'nature' for fear of destroying an order which started before us, which goes beyond us and which we must not in any way question. Idolising nature in this way we become incapable of undertaking projects for our own good – and I mean responsible projects which enhance human life.

The story of electricity production in Austria illustrates this non-interventionist process. We don't build a nuclear power plant because we don't trust nuclear power. So perhaps we should build a hydro-electric plant? No, because we would have to raze a forest. So let's have a coal-fired plant. But this would pollute the air. So we finish up buying power produced either in nuclear, coal-fired, oil-fired or hydro-electric plants – but from abroad.

And where is this original nature we want to defend and not interfere with? Certainly not in Europe, except for a couple of mountain tops – and so many climbers have been there I am not even sure about that! The 'original nature' we talk about in Europe was fashioned by human beings; it has not been 'original' for a very long time.

## Modern Nature

The second concept of nature came out of the Renaissance, a time when man shuffled off his God-given destiny in a divine and hierarchical world to become master of nature's destiny. This is a very materialist concept of nature, even if it was idealistic philosophers like Descartes who invented it. Nature here is the opposite of man. It is what man is not. For man is intelligence, knowledge, understanding and master of this material world he calls 'Nature'. And he will subject this nature to two things: to knowledge and to the techniques born of this knowledge.

Hence the beginning of the adventurous experiments which had the first scholars of the era condemned by the Church; for they wanted to define the world not in terms of a theology, but in terms of human knowledge, through science. They saw themselves as physically part of nature, but separated from it by their minds. And so, trying to reduce nature to lines and curves or sets of calculations, they discovered the great laws of physics and mathematics, and so paved the way for modern science. This is the history of science as we know it today, with its apotheosis in the triumphant positivism of the nineteenth century – to reduce the complex to the simplest, and nature to a set of mathematical laws the mind can analyse and then synthesise.

This second concept of nature is more 'modern' than the first, but its great disadvantage is the notion of the scientist it created, and the engineer mentality which this scientist spawned. Today's engineers, when faced with the task of planning a route for a road or railway line, for example, do not start by going onto the land and following in the steps of human experience. They do not have the richness and diversity of the land in their heads when they trace their lines first on paper, then on maps. They have the shortest, quickest, surest route in their heads. Only after do they go onto the land.

Because for them, nature is pure space they have to work with, and not a living, breathing environment. It only becomes that if it interferes with or facilitates the carrying through of their project.

The problem of a political approach to environment is that both concepts of nature have to be taken into account and a balance has to be struck between the need to graft human projects onto the environment and the need to preserve the richness of that environment.

A Minister of Environment studying the plans for a new motorway will have to face an association which argues that the motorway will cross a wetland, thereby destoying the habitats of so many plant and animal species. The engineer in charge of the project will say that if they circumvent the land in question, the motorway will be longer and will cost so much more. Both positions represent human needs. The task for the politician is to strike a balance between the two.

## What is a man?

If we can ask ourselves what nature is and how we should respect it, then should we not also ask what man is, and whether our own inventions, progress and development respect human potential and richness. In one way, human development can be seen in terms of simple evolution, needs, consumption, knowledge and technology. But here there is an important question. Is the logic of this development – shorter travelling time, more communication, more energy, more food and more waste – not a series of mechanisms, each engendering the next? (We can make jet engines that go faster and further, so we hold conferences further away, etc.) Or is there a meaning, a line of thought, or a choice which gives direction to and fuels this development?

Some examples would tend to prove the first viewpoint. The high-speed TGV train (*Train à Grande Vitesse*) is a remarkable invention which shortens travelling time enormously. But at a time when France was, and still is, trying to hand over more power and independence to the regions, and to reduce the centralisation and concentration in the capital with all the bureaucratic slowness these entail and the awful quality of life they engender for the inhabitants – at such a time, the TGV system was set up to carry passengers from the provinces to Paris and back again, and not from provincial city to provincial city. Why? Because the meaning of this technology for human development was not thought through. The quickest and shortest answer was applied.

Another example followed the accident at the Union Carbide plant at Bhopal, where 2,000 people were killed and several tens of thousands were injured. The chemical produced there, methyl isocyanate (MIC), was also being manufactured in a factory in southern France. As Minister of the Environment, I wanted to see the safety measures at this factory. The team of engineers I took with me to the plant explained the movement of the chemicals from one section to another and I tried to see – as an outsider – if I could not see a fault in the system anywhere.

Afterwards, in a meeting with local inhabitants, plant workers and local councillors, precisely because I was not an engineer, I naïvely asked the question of what the MIC manufactured here was used for. Several people did not know. The management did, and told me that it was a pesticide used against a little worm which attacks sugar beet. I admit I was shocked. This very dangerous chemical is being manufactured around the world to give us a better yield of sugar beet so that we can produce more surplus sugar and feed more surplus cattle and make the sugar and beef mountains we have in Europe even bigger! So why is this product manufactured? Simply because it sells and makes profits. The mad logic of economics.

## Environment and the quality of life

As a politician I often hear other politicians talking of their successes or failures. More often than not the criteria for their assessment are whether money was made or lost – what the effect on the balance of payments was. Politics today has been reduced to economics. We discuss wealth, systems of production and progress in technology, but leave out one fundamental question: 'What are we producing and why?'

If we wish to think about the considerations we need to bear in mind when drafting laws, for example in environment, we must not just contain the damage or indicate the risks. This is what Ministers of Environment tend to do when they meet: to look into how we can reduce the amount of such and such a gas in the air, or avoid the destruction of the ozone layer by banning aerosol sprays. But we do not ask ourselves, for example, why advertising constantly bombards us with the merits of such products. Unfortunately all this is part of the way things are, of making money, of economics, of all those things whose meaning we do not talk about enough.

One of these things is work. Not the type which interests economists and politicians – the saleable work producing wages and profits. But all the other 'work' or activities that we humans do – many of which are carried out by women: education, organising daily routines, caring for the young and elderly and so on. We need to think about a good economic policy that would reorganise the working week so that we might avoid overtiredness and stress, and in so doing perhaps help alleviate the unemployment that blights so many countries.

This concerns the quality of life. Choking on the exhaust fumes of a car in front of us is no worse than choking in a society where we feel worthless or out of place, and where our wives, or husbands, or sons, or neighbours are suffering from the threat of heart disease or any other illness because work is badly distributed and organised.

When I was appointed Minister of the Environment in France, I asked to have the double title of Minister of Environment and Quality of Life. I do not think I furthered the quality of life very much in France. Yet at least I tried not to think of the environment as plant life, animal life and life on earth without man, but rather as everything that surrounds us as human beings – our natural habitat in the biological sense, our urban habitat and the framework of our leisure and social activities.

Chapter 23

# The ozone layer and climatic change

by Mustafa Tolba

The 'Montreal Protocol' to limit the emissions of the CFC family of chemicals and of the halons[1] which are damaging the ozone layer was an historic decision for three reasons. Signed in September 1987, it is

(1) the first truly global agreement on protection of the environment;
(2) the first global *pre-emptive* environmental agreement: it looks ahead to face a distant threat and enables action to be taken now to prevent grave damage in the future;
(3) a precedent for further global action against global dangers to the environment.

The agreement required a decade of gradually intensifying work by scientists, diplomats, lawyers, and politicians with the United Nations Environment Programme (UNEP) involved in the entire process. The story serves as a classic example of how UNEP carries out its mandate to catalyse and co-ordinate actions to protect and improve the global environment.

---

[1] CFCs are chlorofluorocarbons. Halons are compounds related to CFCs having bromine rather than chlorine as their halogenated component; they are used primarily as fire suppressants.

Ozone, a form of oxygen, is a pungent, colourless gas.[2] Ozone concentrations at ground level are normally very low – fortunately, because ozone is extremely poisonous. However, above the earth ozone is a blessing. Life on earth depends on this thin veil because ozone acts as a kind of sponge, absorbing ultraviolet radiation from the sun, shielding the earth from the most harmful radiation. But even at the low levels now reaching the Earth radiation causes skin cancer and eye damage. If more radiation penetrates, the impact on human health, agriculture, plants, marine life, and climate could be very great. Hence the importance of preserving the ozone layer.

In 1974, US scientists suggested that CFCs, commonly used for domestic and industrial purposes, rise to the stratosphere and cause a catalytic reaction which destroys ozone. In 1976, the Governing Council of UNEP directed that this possible threat to the global environment be investigated. The next year UNEP convened a meeting of experts who adopted a twenty-one point Plan of Action on the Ozone Layer and gave UNEP the role and responsibility of collating, disseminating and encouraging research.

At that stage there was no prima facie case against CFCs, but already some governments were very anxious. In 1976, Canada had announced it would order the progressive elimination of CFC-11 and CFC-12 and would prohibit their use in non-essential aerosols (spray cans). In 1978, the United States government prohibited the use of CFCs as propellants in aerosol containers.

Investigation of the extent, composition and photochemistry of the ozone layer continued. Between 1977 and 1985 UNEP published seven separate assessments of the severity of the threat to the ozone layer. Then in 1984–85 there came a scientific bombshell.

Measurements taken in the Antarctic spring (September–October) of 1984 and historical records compiled by the British Antarctic Survey combined to show that the ozone layer over the Antarctic had been declining sharply since the late 1970s. Moreover, the data revealed that since 1957 there had been recurrent annual depletion of some forty per cent of the layer each spring, followed by a recovery to normal levels in the summer.

As a result UNEP convened the Vienna Conference of March 1985 which committed governments to 'take appropriate measures to protect human health and the environment' from the adverse effects of human activities which are likely to modify the ozone layer. On the basis of scientific observations and warnings, the community of nations decided to act in advance and not to wait for the absolute proof of cause and effect that might come too late to avoid irreparable harm.

---

2 Oxygen = $O_2$; ozone = $O_3$.

Pressures for global regulations and limitations to reduce emissions of CFCs were also growing, despite the great commercial interests involved. Global production of CFCs is worth over US$ 2 billion a year and CFCs form the basic material of other industrial products worth billions more. It is noteworthy that the leaders of the chemical industry contributed invaluable technical data essential for making the decisions on how to protect the ozone layer.

The crucial scientific meeting came in April 1987, when UNEP convened scientists from Europe and the United States. Their conclusions were the basis of the Montreal agreement. Their main conclusion was that the rate of ozone depletion depends on the control strategy. They agreed that with no control the ozone layer may be modified to an extent which will certainly increase human cancers and will probably affect agricultural production, atmospheric pollution and climate change. They concluded that only stringent controls, equivalent to a true global freeze of present emissions of all potential ozone-destroying chemicals, could save the ozone layer from serious depletion.

The September 1987 Montreal agreement will mean a reduction by fifty per cent in the consumption of the damaging chemicals by 1999. There may be a case for stricter regulations sooner. The agreement is flexible enough to permit further limitations if there is scientific evidence for them. That is now accumulating. UNEP retains the machinery to consider it, for the Agreement obliges UNEP to continue its role in the issue of protection of the ozone layer.

## The greenhouse effect

The precedent of the ozone accord may open the way for a global response to another environmental threat – modification of the climate, the global warming or 'greenhouse effect'.

Mankind has now replaced nature as the engine of climatic change. The changing atmosphere is now a consequence of human actions in destroying forests, burning fossil fuels, and the uncontrolled emission of waste gases to the atmosphere. The 'outer limit' of the climate – the limit to which it can be stressed before permanent alteration occurs – has been reached. The accumulation of carbon dioxide, chlorofluorocarbons and other radiatively active trace gases in the air is such that global temperatures have now risen above the norm. Acid rain and accumulation of toxic pollutants are other results.

All geographical regions and all environmental sectors are likely to be affected, to a greater or lesser degree, by climate change. The social and economic well-being of all people on earth may be severely disrupted. The basic estimations, most generally and most recently agreed, are as follows:

If greenhouse gases continue to be emitted at projected rates, then their concentration in the atmosphere will double by the early part of the next century. This could result in global mean temperatures rising by between 1.5°C and 4.5°C in the next thirty to forty years. During the same period thermal expansion of the ocean and, to some extent, glacier melt may raise ocean levels by up to one metre.

Even a modest rise in sea level will inundate coastal wetlands and recreational beaches, threaten storm barriers, salinate reservoirs and water treatment plants in estuaries, and threaten habitation and livelihood. A one metre rise is calculated to result in the dislocation of fifteen million people in Bangladesh, as much as ten million people in Egypt, and comparable numbers elsewhere. A minimum cost of one million dollars per kilometre of coastline, and two billion dollars for each coastal city, are modest estimates of preventive costs that could be required to cope with climate change impacts.

Changes in global atmospheric and ocean circulation and changes in regional rainfall patterns will occur in ways presently impossible to predict with confidence. Such changes are beginning now and will continue through the next century unless action is taken to stabilise the atmosphere. But so far virtually no specific actions are being taken to stabilise, limit, delay or mitigate the changes. It is a matter of urgency to develop and agree on strategies for an effective global response.

Climate change cannot be prevented; however, it may be possible to limit its extent, delay its onset and take actions to alleviate the worst effects. To do this it is necessary to gain a better understanding of the problem and for nations to agree on and implement national, regional and global measures.

UNEP has a mandate to encourage the formulation of response options and the development of a co-ordinated global policy. The need for action is urgent, but because of the still limited understanding of the problem, particularly of the effects of climatic change, the priority is to improve scientific knowledge.

Despite extensive research, most scientists say they will not be able to predict future regional climates with any degree of confidence without fifteen more years of research. And without accurate scenarios of regional climate impacts, analyses can only border on the speculative. There are more uncertainties about human socio-economic consequences. Energy conservation and technological remedies to reduce emissions need to be applied soon if they are to be effective. Adaptive strategies – for instance sea defences and water engineering projects – must be designed to be effective in the climate of the twenty-first century and to cope with the climatic 'shocks' which may characterise the transition from one climatic regime to another.

The scale of UNEP's co-ordinating work is limited by the human and financial resources available. To overcome this restriction, we are trying to encourage the widest possible participation in addressing the issues. But although it is desirable to wait for internationally co-ordinated scientific assessments, a range of policy options and strategies must be developed and examined now.

The main thrusts of UNEP's programme of action on climate change caused by changes in the atmosphere are:

- to arrange for internationally accepted assessments of climate change and its impacts;
- to develop and test policy options to limit or delay climate change – or to adapt to the change once it has begun;
- to facilitate dialogue between the scientific community and policy makers on the impacts of climate change and on the development of policy response alternatives;
- to increase the level of public information on the issue; and
- to co-ordinate international action on studies of the impacts of climate variability and change.

A similar and complementary programme will identify and address the impacts of climate change on sensitive sectors of the environment: health, water resources, sea levels, marine and terrestrial ecosystems, etc.

Another important role for UNEP is co-ordination of international activities on the environment. Several countries have climate impact programmes, others have impact groups operating independently. Many countries are not carrying out climate impact research at all or are doing so in an uncoordinated manner. UNEP is establishing a network of the more active climate impact programmes and facilitating communication and co-operation among them. Expansion of the network will increase as more countries are drawn in. All of the special task forces and programmes constituted by UNEP to address the issue of climate change will be working throughout the next decade – and perhaps into the next century – in one form or another. For some specialists and scientists, this issue may become a life's work – for the sake of the life of all on our planet.

In informing the public of the latest developments in shaping responses to the challenge of climate change, UNEP also seeks the public's continued attention and support. It will be a long task for all of us, but it is a task in which we must not falter if we are to leave to future generations in the next century a world in which human beings can live in health and harmony with the environment.

Chapter 24

# Environment and health in the light of WHO's mandate

by Wilfried Kreisel

In May 1977, the World Health Assembly – WHO's supreme policy-making body – took a momentous decision. It resolved that the main social target of governments and WHO in the coming decades should be the attainment by all the people of the world by the year 2000 of a level of health that will permit them to lead a socially and economically productive life.

This policy, popularly known as *Health for All by the Year 2000*, has pointed to the environment at large as a major determinant of human health. Moreover, it has highlighted the need for WHO to extend its efforts beyond the traditionally orientated medical programmes – both curative and preventive – to a broader approach to health policy through an emphasis on primary health care and on man's environment and its relationship with health.

## Safe water and sanitation

Threats to human health from environmental hazards – such as vectors[1], parasites, bacteria and viruses that frequently stem from the absence of hygienically safe water and adequate sanitation facilities – still pose the

1 An organism that transmits a specific cause of a disease.

main public health concerns in developing countries. In addition, pollution via air, land, water, food, energy development, and the adverse effects of human, agricultural and industrial activity add an increasingly alarming dimension to human health and environmental concerns. Society is being exposed to more 'insults' to health than in previous centuries.

In the evolution of society from simplicity to complexity, man has had an amazing capacity to confront these threats and to create control devices for their prevention, but most often belatedly and too often unsuccessfully. While we profit immeasurably from advances in science and technology, we pay an increasing penalty for them.

For example, in the huge industrial part of Kaohsiung on the south-western coast of Taiwan, the number of factories increased from 5,623 to 62,474, between 1950 and 1980. The fastest rate of increase was by the factories producing hazardous wastes: plastics, chemicals, petroleum refining, pesticides, leather tanning. Taiwan's air is so polluted that for 17 per cent of the year it is officially considered harmful to health. In 1988, only one per cent of Taiwan's human excrement is subject to primary sewage treatment, and Taiwan has the world's highest incidence of hepatitis B.[2]

The key lies in recognising the penalties of modern technology and in creating institutional machinery to control, modify or eliminate them. The best managerial device has not yet been discovered. Should the approach be educational, investigative, arbitrary – or adversarial and punitive? A new strategy is needed.

Basic needs that have not concerned a majority of the world's population for more than a century are still the main determinant of the health status in the developing world. Despite significant and ongoing progress (aided by the momentum created by the International Drinking Water Supply and Sanitation Decade ) more than 50 per cent of the world's rural population lacks water supply and 84 per cent lacks any type of sanitation facility. More than one-third of the five billion people on earth live in an unsafe environment: they have no access to safe water or sanitation *and* they have poor shelter and often an insufficient food supply.

The widespread diseases associated with such poor facilities represent more than half of the mortality and up to three-quarters of the morbidity figures in developing countries. These figures include not only schistosomiasis (200 million people infected) and diarrhoea (1 billion episodes per year with a resulting figure of 5 million deaths), but also debilitating diseases such as guinea worm (1 million cases every year), trachoma, intestinal parasites, and dental and skeletal fluorosis. This is why WHO's Environmental Health Programme still allocates about one-

---

2 *The Economist*, March 1988.

third of its budgetary resources to community water supply and sanitation activities.

## Consequences of global and local pollution

Populations in developing countries are also affected by the consequences of global and local pollution which are no longer confined to the industrialized world. In the majority of developing countries, pollution problems are second in environmental priority to major challenges such as soil conservation, desertification, and environmental health issues related to water-borne and fecal-borne diseases. But this is only because the major challenges are so serious.

Ten out of the sixteen cities in the world that exceed the WHO guideline values for air quality are third world countries. Contamination of groundwater with nitrates, safe handling of pesticides, and disposal of hazardous wastes are increasing concerns for public health administrators throughout the world. There is anxiety about the acute effects to people's health from exposure to hazardous wastes containing toxic chemicals at concentrations high enough to cause immediate harm.

But perhaps the most important problem with hazardous wastes arises from the potential they have at low concentrations to contaminate the human environment. In the long term we may be creating a deadly time bomb. How large are the natural assimilative capacities of the environment and the biological variabilities of the human organism to cope over long periods with the chronic effects of exposure to low-level toxic substances? This is a question for which a clear answer is not possible at present.

Among the many WHO programmes that deal with the problems of hazardous waste the work of the International Programme on Chemical Safety (IPCS), is of particular importance. Co-sponsored by the ILO and UNEP,[3] the programme's primary mandate is to conduct and disseminate evaluations of the health and environmental risks of chemicals of priority concern. The programme's aim is to assist governments in setting health-based standards and in initiating preventive or control measures.

The IPCS evaluations are conducted by international groups of experts and the results are presented in environmental health criteria documents and in different types of health and safety guides and cards. The programme has already made available evaluated information for nearly 70 priority chemicals, with more in various stages of completion. The evaluations contain confirmation on sources, routes of exposure and observed effects on

---

3 The International Labour Organization (ILO) and the United Nations Environment Programme (UNEP).

health and the environment. Whenever the information allows, they also include recommendations as to the 'no effect' or safe levels of the chemicals.

If the hazardous waste problem is to be dealt with adequately, we must steadily build up capacities for environmental health hazard control at *each* national level. This is the *raison d'être* of WHO's technical co-operation programme. Its activities are carried out by the six WHO Regional Offices in collaboration with the Member States and involve the training of staff; the development of legislation, regulations and standards; the strengthening of laboratory and monitoring capabilities; and the promotion of inter-sectoral action for environmental and health protection.

Urbanisation and the whole range of problems associated with this totally artificial environment pose even more complex risks to human health through environmental hazards. Cities face the whole list of problems mentioned above, plus specific ones resulting from the concentration of huge population densities on limited land. Urban concentrations and the rapidly growing proportion of the world's population living in cities demand a revision of the traditional approach towards environmental health.

## The need for a comprehensive approach

The new concept that is emerging is a comprehensive approach, encompassing all the social, economic, and environmental factors conducive to health within the framework of a global programme of health promotion. Thus the new WHO approach includes all the physical and chemical factors which have been part of its environmental programme since the organisation was founded. But it also includes the promotion of suitable housing, safe processing of food, dietary patterns conducive to health, and changing lifestyles to reduce the burden of accidents and the toll of cancer and cardiovascular diseases.

The perception that the careful management of our living environment is a basic condition for preserving a level of health, which in turn ensures, among other things, the sustainability of development efforts and the sustainability of a socially and economically productive life, has become one of the major driving forces behind the WHO programme. The Health Promotion programme developed by the Regional Office for Europe, the Healthy Cities movement, and many other initiatives participate in this endeavour. The long-term National Programme of Health Promotion, submitted last November to the Parliament of Hungary, is an example that clearly reflects this renewed attitude towards environmental health as the cornerstone for all improvements of health status during the coming decades.

This new approach goes beyond traditional environmental technology. It leads to the destruction of barriers between well-established disciplines and specialisations. It raises queries about our own behaviour. We at WHO are convinced that the appropriate response to the challenges of the next century depends upon our ability to break down the barriers between old categories and upon our ability to convince our contemporaries of the need for action.

The World Commission on Environment and Development entreated governments, multilateral and bilateral financing institutions and the United Nations system to review their policies, programmes and budgets with a view to contributing to sustainable development – a development which allows future generations to continue to live a viable life on spaceship earth. It is a call that cannot be ignored.

Chapter 25

# Environment policy in the European Communities

by Laurens Jan Brinkhorst

The issue of the quality of life is a basic component and part of the future of the European Community as we near the end of the twentieth century. If we compare the situation of 1988 with 1973, when the Community's first environmental action programme had just begun, one very basic difference is that the question is no longer *whether* there should be a European environmental policy, but rather *what kind* of European environmental policy?

In 1973 the European Community (EC) was seen basically as an economic instrument, with limited goals, customs tariffs and the like. Environment seemed a secondary issue – if that. Now, in 1988, the battle has been won: environmental policy is firmly anchored in the Treaty of Rome, the EC Constitution, through the first substantial modification since the treaty's adoption in 1958.

The first two environmental action programmes, launched in 1973 and 1977, were largely concerned with seeking immediate answers to pollution problems, but their wide ranging and far-sighted approach provided the basis for Community environment policy to date. The third programme in 1983 introduced an overall strategy for the protection of the environment and natural resources, and recognised that to take environmental considerations into account at the early stages makes sound economic and environmental sense. In short, it showed that prevention is better – and more cost effective – than cure.

These three programmes have made considerable achievements: more than 100 directives have been introduced into the laws of the EC member states. There has been particular success in the control of discharges of dangerous substances into water, the control of chemicals – both on the market and in industry – and the protection of nature. But the European environment still continues to deteriorate; new efforts are needed.

The European Community's fourth environmental action programme, officially adopted at the end of October 1987, will run until 1992. The preventive approach of the previous programme is continued, but there is particular emphasis on *integrating* that approach into all other sectors of activity. Environmental protection is recognised as an essential element of any economic, industrial, agricultural or social policy.

The programme also sets out a number of priority themes which will be the subject of specific proposals over the coming years. These include air and water pollution, the control of chemicals, the protection of the soil, the disposal and recycling of waste, the conservation of natural resources, developments in biotechnology, and the safe use of nuclear power. This indicates that European environmental policy is now an integral component of the European scene.

## A different viewpoint

A second basic difference between 1973 and 1988 is, that in societal terms, we now look at environment in a very different way. In the 1960s, unparalleled economic growth went hand in hand with unparalleled destruction of the environment. We swept behind cupboards and under carpets whatever fall-out of the economic process took place.

The early 1970s saw the pendulum swing to the other side. We had the philosopy of 'zero growth' and the idea that the only way to save the environment was to forget about economic growth. I think both those positions have now been proven fallacious. In the 1980s we are in the midst of an historically new concept. We realise that economic growth is necessary, certainly vital as far as the Third World countries are concerned. We also recognise that there will be no hope of saving the environment unless economic growth takes place. But at the same time there is the fundamental realisation that the ecology is the absolutely necessary foundation of that growth. The World Commission on Environment and Development chaired by Prime Minister Gro Harlem Brundtland, last year underlined the concept of 'sustainable development' as a particular element of that overall orientation.

The third difference that I see is that the European Community in the early 1970s was a different animal than it is today. We have always had a basic differentiation between the north and the south, but Europeans now have to learn to combat environment issues on a continental scale. That is very difficult for us, emmeshed as we all are in provincial nets of nationalism.

When I am in the Federal Republic of Germany, I hear many bad things about European environmental policy because the issue of car emissions and acid rain is at stake. But I do not hear anybody saying that the Federal Republic of Germany is the biggest polluter in industrial terms – not because it is any worse than anybody else, but because it is the major industrialized country in the Community.

When I speak in my own country, the Netherlands, the Dutch are very proud about their environmental consciousness, but nobody tells me that the Dutch are the worst polluters in agricultural terms. There are five times more animals per hectare in the Netherlands than on average in any country of the Community. The pile of manure produced every year by Dutch farms corresponds to a string of trucks which can encircle the world; and every year the process repeats itself.

My point is not to attack any individual country – certainly not the Federal Republic of Germany, and certainly not the Netherlands. But I do wish to make clear that as far as environmental pollution is concerned, *all* Europeans are sinners and we must realise that there is a necessity to look at individual issues as they come along.

This immediately brings me to the fourth major difference between the start of the First Action Programme and today: that is the context in which the Directorate General for the Environment, for which I am responsible, has to operate. One cannot disassociate environmental issues from national, industrial and agricultural interests. It is no longer good enough to point to the threat to the environment and mobilise public opinion in a general way. Practical solutions will only stick if we find solutions which can be implemented in specific terms and are supported by those who are directly affected. Now that environment has finally 'come of age' as a major policy area, we have to have a more sophisticated and mature approach, proposing realistic policies that will take the various distinctions and interests into account, while at the same time continuing to lead the way forward to protect our vital resources and recover our position from the damage we have done in the past.

## The relevance of the European framework

These, I think, are the essential differences, the background between 1988 and the beginning of the 1970s. It is clear that the European framework has become much more essential, because we now realise that we have to overcome the 'provincial' nationalistic attitudes of states in order to have a more comprehensive European – and in some areas global – approach to environmental issues. One might ask, of course, to what extent is the European framework relevant? *Why* is the EEC an organism which potentially can be effective in combatting pollution and which in general can help promote the environment?

I would say firstly because the environment policy, based in the Community Treaty, is now an integral part of the other EC policies, like the internal market, the industrial policy, and the common agricultural policy. In today's world an effective environmental policy *must* be integrated with the other components of public policy, as Dr Bernatzky and Mr Häussler point out in relation to urban planning and the role of housing.

Secondly, the European Community is the only major international organisation which has a real, effective legislative and administrative framework and legal capacity in the field of environment. Therefore, in order to avoid issues like distortion of competition when setting environmental standards – an important element for any industry and any actor in the industrial scene – one must have policies of a European nature.

Thirdly, through the Commission, the EC's administrative arm, *decision-making takes place in an even broader framework than a strictly inter-governmental one.* If it is true that environmental interests and environmental priorities in each individual country are closely linked with national industrial or agricultural priorities, then some kind of balancing mechanism, some kind of initiating role is needed in order to put these various issues and interests in a proper, broader European perspective. I claim that this is the essential role which the Commission of the European Communities can and must play. No environmental policies have been adopted by the Council of Ministers without initiatives by the Commission.

Fourthly, and very importantly, the European Community is the only international organisation which represents the beginning of a democratic framework, of a supranational government. I believe that, as far as the environment is concerned, the only effective pressure group is you and me – the individual members of the public. It is not industry; it is not agriculture; it is *none* of the other pressure groups. It is the general public.

This position has a strength and a weakness. The weakness is that environmental policy affects all of us, but it affects all of us in very different ways, and we all play different roles. In one case we act as a consumer, in another case as a trade-union member, in another case as an employee, and in yet another case as a taxpayer. That is why, by and large, environmental policies are very often less effective than they could be. But at the same time we are there as members of the general public.

The strength of this position is that the general public is indeed realising more and more that we are on the way to forever undermining our own environment. Issues like the ozone layer and the greenhouse effect are simply fundamental demonstrations of that point. The *Eurobarometer* survey published in January 1988 indicated how high on the list of public concerns and priorities environmental issues now are. One question asked was: 'What is the task for a European government, in case there should be a European government?' On the list, environment had to compete with monetary affairs, defence, and other issues which are dear to all of our hearts – like problems of unemployment and inflation. But, for the first time ever on the Eurobarometer, environment was among the top three.

### *Global concern*

My final point on the relevance of the European framework is that many of our environmental issues have become of global concern. If one wants to have an effective environmental policy, there must be international negotiations on issues like the ozone layer and chlorofluorocarbons (CFCs). The main producers of CFCs are the Europeans, the Americans, the Japanese and the Russians.

I was one of the participants in Montreal in September 1987 when the nations of the world discussed the ozone layer protocol and I was struck by the fact that in the discussions between them there was no ideology at stake. There was nothing of the traditional East-West competition; there was very little of the traditional North-South division. But there *was* very much of the issue of equality of treatment of industry, such as adaptation periods and so on. Now my claim would be that *if* the European Community had been (as usual) in 'ordre dispersé' and in very different frameworks – with the Germans different from the Dutch, and the French different from the Italians – we would not have been able to play any role at all in Montreal. And that would have occurred in a situation where the Europeans are the largest producers of CFCs in the world – accounting for fifty per cent of the total – and at the same time the largest exporters.

## Three issues for the future

While I hope I have made a thoroughly convicing case for the relevance of the European framework in environmental policy, I wish also to point out frankly that everything which is done in the European framework is not so beautiful. Despite the fact that we now have environment embedded in the Treaty of Rome, I think the Community still has to prove the effectiveness, the efficiency and the drive which should underlie our environmental policy. There are three issues upon which we should concentrate.

The first is the issue of execution and implementation of existing European environmental policies. Since the beginning of the 1970s we have introduced more than 100 directives into the legal structures of member states. These directives are binding legislation but they are indirect legislation as they must be incorporated by the member states into their national legislation. They are similar to the legislation which the federal parliament enacts in the Federal Republic of Germany and which then has to be executed at Länder level. As such, it is quasi-federal legislation. But unfortunately, since 1973, the environmental directives have moved to third place on the list of those directives for which the Commission has initiated infringement proceedings against the member states for failure to implement – directly after those on agriculture, the internal market and industrial affairs. I can assure you, as Director-General of this department, that this is not a very happy position to be in!

It is absolutely essential that in the future we place a higher priority on proper implementation, not only for the sake of implementing the legislation concerned, but also because basically the non-observance of *any* law erodes the credibility of a society. So both the Community and the member states must do better, for both have been at fault. For the last fifteen years the Commission has concentrated perhaps too much on being simply a legislation machine, constantly producing new proposals. Now we must also concentrate on the issue of implementation.

Member states still very often lack the political will to implement Community law. They hide behind traditional concepts of a lack of scientific evidence to justify some of the directives. Here I would like to invoke the view of His Royal Highness, Prince Charles, who has repeatedly spoken on the subject. If we have to wait until scientific evidence provides the final proof that CFCs, for instance, can affect the ozone layer, it would be like asking a surgeon to operate after the patient has died. I hope that public pressure will help to combat this traditional view that 100 per cent scientific proof is a prerequisite before any environmental measure can be taken.

The second issue on which the Environment Directorate should now concentrate was under discussion at the end of February 1988 in an informal EC Council meeting in Bavaria. The issue on the table was Agriculture and Environment. This was the first time that an EC Environmental Council met informally to discuss rather than to dispute a problem, and to analyse jointly rather than to compromise.

The situation is that since 1973, in relative terms, industrial pollution in the industrialized world has gone down. There is now an awareness, and I think a great readiness, on the part of industry to combat pollution, despite the fact that problems like time limits and issues of competition among the Americans, Europeans, and Japanese continue. Yet paradoxically, the agricultural environment in the European Community is worse in 1988 than in 1973.

This is not simply the fault of the farmers, who at the present time are reacting very defensively, and understandably so. In the past they have been told that they should produce more; they have been told that there should be more pesticides; they have been told that there are many developments which can actually help to increase their income. Now they are being told just the reverse. They cannot produce more, they must produce less. They cannot use more pesticides, they must use less pesticides. The result is that farmers do not want to even talk about taking extra environmental measures now.

But this informal Environmental Council meeting in Bavaria came to just the opposite conclusion: the ministers said that it is precisely the right moment to take measures and to start a reasonable dialogue between the environmentalists and the farmers. Interestingly, the environment ministers came to this conclusion just as the European Year of the Environment (EYE) drew to its close.

As far as EYE is concerned, the Commission feels the year was useful in many ways. Firstly, it has certainly sensitised the European population even more to the urgent need for effective environmental measures.

Secondly, it has 'Europeanized' the environmental debate. The EYE has taken us out of our parochial roles of individual nations by demonstrating that obvious environmental issues are either very different or differently perceived in every country. It has therefore created the background and understanding for better policies and the possibilities for Europeans to act jointly.

Thirdly, it has demonstrated the inadequacy of current environmental policy, including the issue of implementation. And finally, the European Year of the Environment gave us a chance to continue after March 1988. The show is not over; it has just begun.

# Part IV

# The Artists and the Philosophers

Chapter 26

# Modern art and the psychology of an age

by René Huyghe

Max Ernst – the great Surrealist – said in 1950: 'We have to exclude all conscious mental thinking from the origins of the work to reach total inspiration. ... the objects of our love and hate appear on the canvas without our willing contribution. The artist just has to fix them there.'

Psychoanalysis – particularly of the Jungian variety – shows us that the images thrown up in our dreams are a direct expression of the depths of our innermost selves. The images thrown out of the artist's imagination express the same thing. For although the essence of a work of art is undoubtedly its esthetic quality, it can reveal much more, and notably the psychology of the artist and through him, the psychology of an age. The study of art from a psychological standpoint can therefore be approached on two levels: we can look at the individual, personal psychology of the artist, or, through what he expresses and how, we can look at the psychology of an era which he suffers or to which he reacts. I shall be taking the latter approach.

## Art and our times

One of the great defects of our age is the predominance of the economic over the spiritual. It is without doubt the fundamental imbalance in our society and that which probably condemns it to decline. The artist, with his

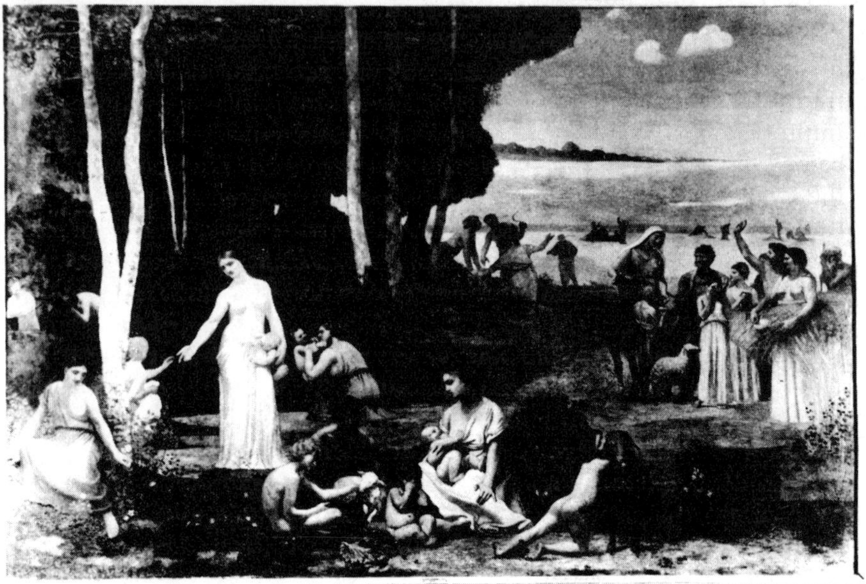

Figure 26.1 Puvis de Chavannes, *L'Eté,* Musée de Chartres

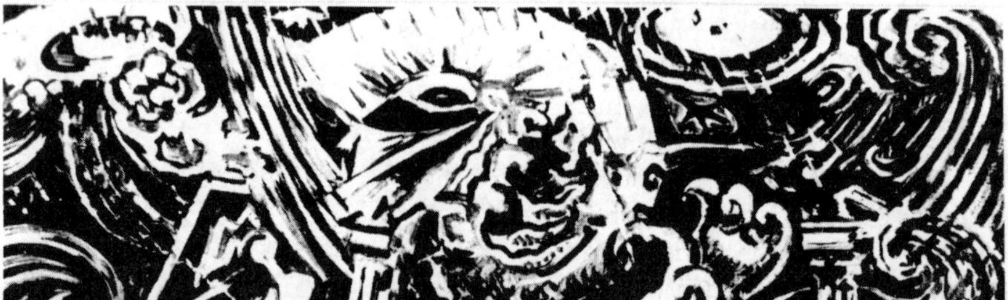

Figure 26.2 André Masson, *Le Fleuve Héraclite*

particular sensibility, has perceived this.

The break with the old perception of civilisation occurred towards the end of the 19th century and a comparison of two works will illustrate this. The first, *L'Eté* ('The Summer') is by Puvis de Chavannes, and is typical of the traditional view of art (Figure 26.1). Painted in 1891, at a time when Impressionism was in full development, it still depicts a world in harmony, balance and security. To realise the extent of the break which took place in the twentieth century, we only need to compare this painting with one by the Surrealist André Masson. Entitled *Le Fleuve Héraclite* ('The Heraclitus river') (Figure 26.2), the remains of the ancient, classical world – a temple, pediments – are toppled, carried away and destroyed by the raging floodtide. All is tumult and disaster.

Until this break then, art generally conveyed the joy of living. Afterwards, it expressed anguish. Another example of this break is the 1881 painting by Auguste Renoir, *Le déjeuner des canotiers* ('The boaters' lunch') which pre-dates Puvis's picture. Everything here is joy and pleasures fulfilled – of life, nature, animals, the sun, love, eating. And yet only eight years later Edvard Munch was to convey the anguish of living. This great Norwegian painter had in fact learned and assimilated Impressionism when he began his career in Paris. But then he went in the opposite direction and his painting *Promenade du Dimanche à Oslo* ('Sunday stroll in Oslo') had two versions which reflect the evolution. The first dates from 1889, and is still very close to Renoir. Well-dressed people leisurely wander about the streets while a band plays – everything captures the joy of living. But three years later he transforms his painting. The main street is still there with the same people in top hats, but now night has fallen and they wander like haggard ghosts, livid and wide-eyed.

Munch went on, in following paintings, to develop his own style – that vision of anguish itself where human beings lose their personalities and individual faces, to become screaming mouths and wide, staring eyes, pursued by unseen deadly figures. And nature is now a torment of sweeping lines and fiery colours.

## Art, man and nature

Let us now look at the problem of the artist faced with the relationship between man and nature. In the middle of the 19th century, in 1854, the great realist, Gustave Courbet painted himself on *Les rochers de Palavas,* ('The rocks of Palavas') facing the sea and infinity. Like Victor Hugo, and all those who believed in the ineluctable march of progress, he was raising his hat to this infinity with a grand gesture, in triumph and with pride. We can compare the same subject dealt with today by the painter Fred Zeller. In

*Ecce homo* the empty beach, sea and sky crush the man, who here and now has become tiny and lost in space, accompanied only by his shadow. (The obsessive fear of our shadow being joined to us has been studied, notably, by the German psychoanalyst, Otto Rank.)

Another symptom of the same malaise is the appearance, in painting and sculpture, of thread-like figures which seem to be eaten away by the space surrounding them. The Belgian painter Spillaert's crushed figures are a good example. The Swiss artist Giacometti, one of the greatest contemporary sculptors, is obsessed by the idea of man being crushed. One striking example is a group of sculptures called *La place de la ville* ('The city square'). Thread-like figures, with excessively thick feet, seem glued to the ground. They can neither move nor communicate between themselves. They do not move towards each other and do not meet. The Swiss critic, Jacques Monnier, reflects: 'To look on this work, we are overcome with dizziness, a dizziness brought on by void, because void seems to be Giocametti's raw material. What is left of man? A character on the edge of nothingness. Taken to its absurd conclusion, surely this culture of the void is despair?' We might think so when we consider the familiar themes of one of the precursors of Surrealism, the Italian Giorgio De Chirico, one of whose paintings is in fact called *Malinconia* ('Melancholy'). The remains of the ancient world rise up out of a deserted space, while in the foreground a woman in black, alone with her shadow, looks overwhelmed with grief.

## The obstacle

So we are both lost in space and crushed by it, we are in a void, alone – except perhaps for our shadow – and are unable to communicate with our fellow humans. We despair. Such are some of the obsessive fears of the contemporary sensibility. The resulting frustration and lack of satisfaction are expressed in modern art and particularly by the image of space being blocked from us by an insurmountable obstacle.

The obstacle has become a sort of unconscious fear and as such is represented in many different schools of art. Max Ernst favoured the theme of the cliff or impenetrable forest, raised up before us. He even combined the two in *La Forêt-arête* ('The edge-forest') in 1927. Nearly sixty years later, a young artist, Reine Mazoyer, conveys space in her landscapes as a series of sterile walls and barriers. And to go back to Fred Zeller again, we see that he has expressed this theme in many of his paintings. In *Nous ne sommes que des images qui passent* ('We are just pictures that pass'), people of all ages sit, overwhelmed with despair, between a quay which plunges behind them and a wall which blocks everything in front. Nature is reduced to the shadow of a tree.

And what about abstract art? By definition, it should not represent anything. But in fact, without knowing it, it very often depicts obstacles. I have chosen three examples. The German Hans Hartung's abstract paintings are nothing other than amazingly barred space. Similarly the figurative American painter, Longdom, in 1949 depicted a space, in *Red City*, which seems to be behind a sort of fence. Elsewhere there are the vague bars of some kind of hedge. In 1976 Simon Hantaï was commissioned to design the poster for an exhibition of modern art. What did he do? He barred space with a criss-cross of spiked wires.

Let us take the opposite of the abstract – Neo-realism. In the Belgian painter Wittewrongel's *Porte* ('Door'), space is blocked out by the door. In Gérald Dareau's 1986 painting *Volet* ('Window blind'), there is a closed window with nailed-down blinds to prevent it being opened. More directly, the artist sometimes depicts human imprisonment. In both the sculptor Ossip Zadkine's *Prisonnière* ('Female prisoner') and Laetitia Hure's *Le Prisonnier* ('The prisoner'), a prisoner desperately puts his or her arms through the bars to try to get free. Zeller once more, always so symptomatic, calls one of his works *Nous sommes tous dans une cage?* ('We are all in a cage?'). Here, not only is a man facing a wall, but on the wall itself we see the shadow of bars.

## Melancholy

It is not surprising, then, that one of the striking themes of our age is melancholy. It is significant that melancholy had already obsessed the late Middle Ages in Northern Europe – when a merchant, bourgeois, positivist civilisation had also pushed out spirituality and fostered imbalance. At that time it was Albrecht Dürer and Lucas Cranach who painted or engraved melancholy. Nearer to our time, Cézanne's *Garçon au gilet rouge* ('Boy in a red waistcoat') is very reminiscent of the clinical pose of the melancholic, as explained by Professor Tellenbach: in a cascade of despondency, the heavy head is supported by the hand, and the elbow is supported by the knee or table. As we enter the twentieth century, we come to Picasso. Painted in 1902 in his 'blue period', *Le vieux Juif* ('The old Jew') sits despondent on the ground. But why blue? Experiments on human volunteers locked up in rooms painted in one colour have shown that while red excites, blue at first soothes, then brings on depression. And the 'blue period' was Picasso's first statement. It is true that he then went through a 'pink period', but this in fact corresponded to a great, but temporary love, and so the change confirms the theory.

Let us look now at the post-First World War generation. In Francis Gruber's *Annonce de l'hiver* ('Winter foreshadowed') (Figure 26.3), we see a

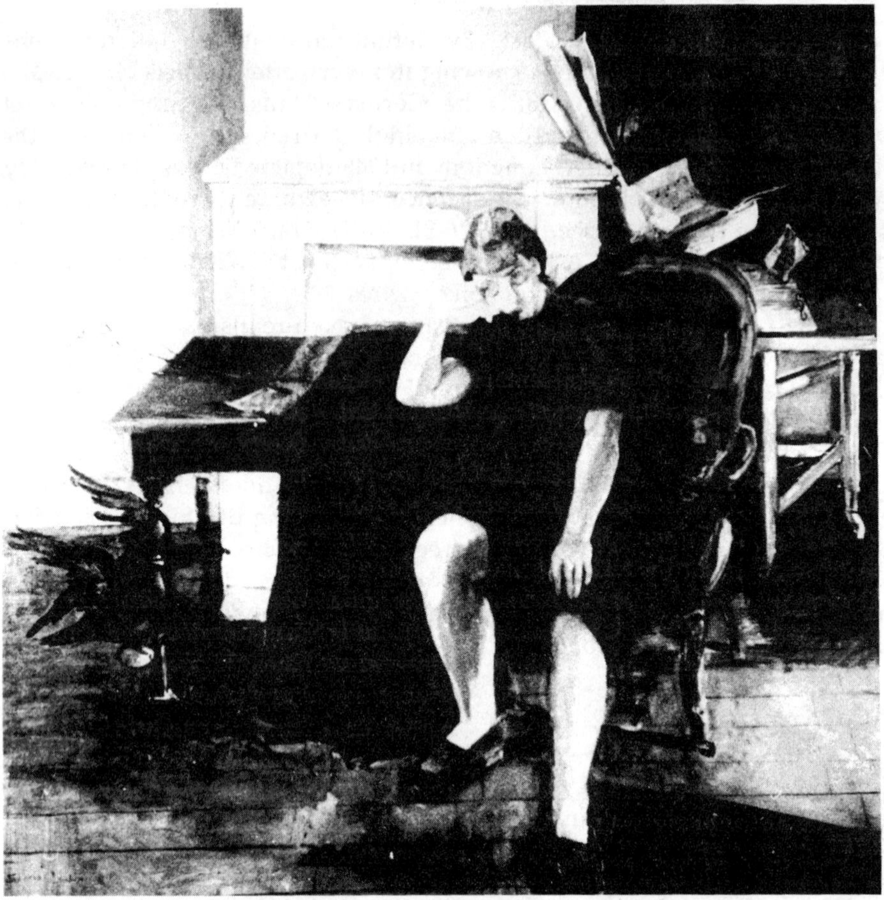

**Figure 26.3 Francis Gruber, *L'Annonce de l'Hiver,* Musée d'Arras**

young woman in the melancholic pose described earlier. All colour has gone. There are birds, but they are dead and stuffed crows. Around is emptiness. Artistic expression was not more optimistic in America. In Edward Hopper's 1926 painting *Solitude, Dimanche après-midi* ('Solitude, Sunday afternoon') the central character sits, world-weary, on the edge of a pavement.

## A scientific explanation: entropy

Can we find a scientific explanation for the evolution in modern art? I believe that we can find in modern art an application of entropy. The second law of thermodynamics states that the quantity of energy in an isolated system remains constant, but disperses progressively and

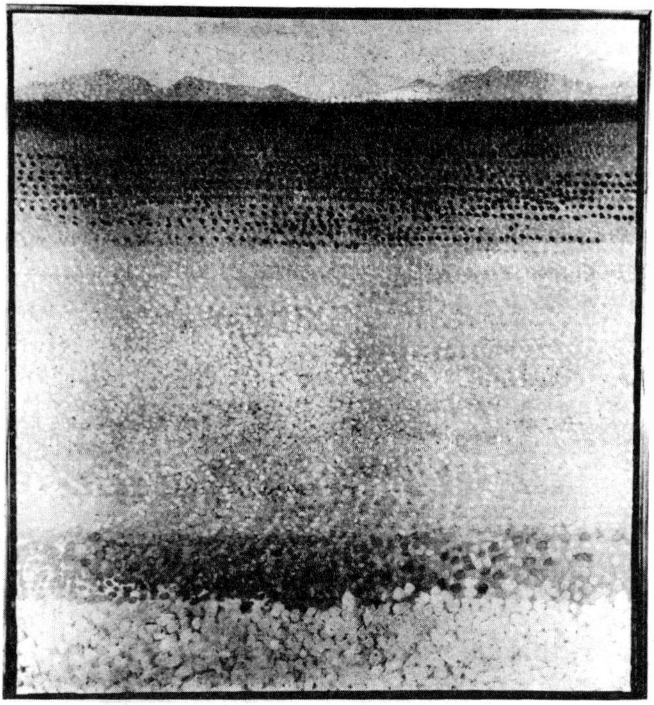

**Figure 26.4 H. Edmond Cross, *Les Iles d'Or*, Musée National d'Art Moderne, Paris**

constantly towards absolute zero. Historians have never thought of looking at the development of contemporary art in this way. And yet in all schools of art, however opposed they are, the typical process of entropy is apparent, a sign that civilisation is exhausting itself.

Let us begin with the Impressionists. What do they do but split up and divide reality into touches of colour, to the extent that Neo-impressionism was called 'pointillism'. In the typical landscape by H. Edmond Cross, *Iles d'Or* ('Islands of gold') (Figure 26.4), we see the emptiness of the beach, the sea and the sky again, but this time broken up and scattered into little, equally-sized dots.

Faced with this danger Cubism reacted. Ordinarily this movement is seen as a return to forms and the problems they pose. But remember that the first cubism was called 'analytical cubism' and that it only came back to forms all the better to break them up or fragment them once again. In Picasso's *L'Homme à la pipe* ('Man with a pipe'), we can recognise the man's moustache, his small beard, the buttons on his waistcoat, his hands on the arms of his armchair and behind him a picture and frame. But everything is broken up, fragmented; what is often overlooked is that Picasso even uses pointillism to colour his surfaces. So Cubism, although a reaction to Impressionism, is subjected to the same law.

And Surrealism? In Yves Tanguy's *Multiplication des Arcs* ('Multiplication of arcs') we find the same sterile dispersion. This time with fragments of bone. Abstract art? The Belgian poet and painter Henri Michaux produced a series of paintings called *Dessins de désagrégation* ('Pictures of disintegration'). The title says all. In my opinion the greatest American abstract artist was Mark Tobey, who died in 1976. All his paintings, like *The universal city* (Figure 26.5), reveal an equal and absolute fragmentation. Looking into the origin of this particular work I discovered that Tobey had taken as his starting point certain non-realist views of

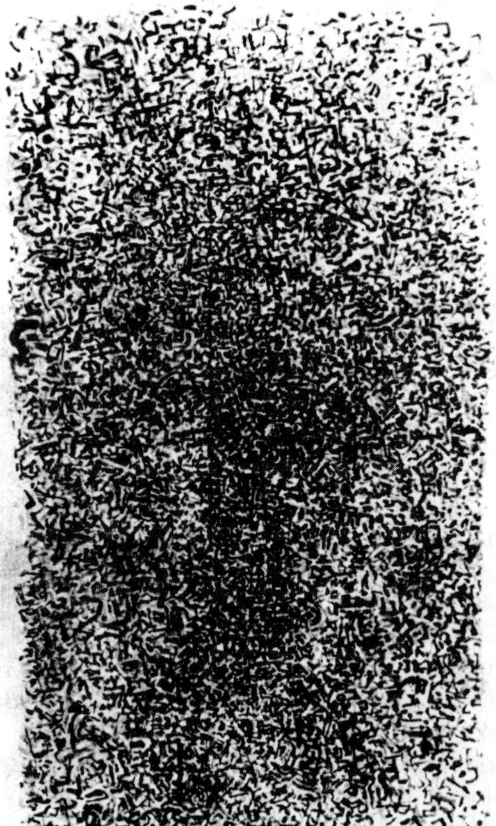

**Figure 26.5 Mark Tobey, *The universal city*, Seattle Art Museum**

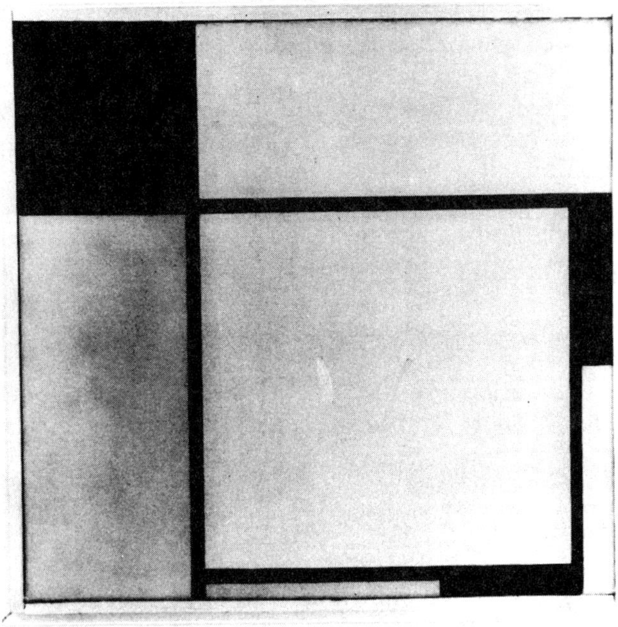

**Figure 26.6 Piet Mondrian,** ***Composition in red, yellow and blue,*** **Guggenheim Museum, New York**

New York he had painted in 1942, like *Broadway*. What was he showing about the modern city? Cars, neon ads and people swarming on the streets – rivalling the stars swarming in the sky. In all these different schools, therefore, we find the same phenomenon resulting from entropy.

## Schizophrenia, Mondrian and Pop Art

But what about Mondrian? Does he not embody the opposite of entropy with his rigorous squares? (Figure 26.6) Here we are faced with another phenomenon. One of the hallmarks of the depression that modern art depicts is schizophrenia. The word itself comes from the Greek 'skhizein', to split, fragment. So it is a parallel to entropy. Dr Dracoulidès, who published a psychoanalysis of Picasso said that 'progressive disintegration is linked to the evolution of his psychopathy'. And Dr Ferdière, studying schizophrenics, asserts that 'cramming' is aimed at filling the void, that void which characterises the world of schizophrenics.' (The logical result of destructiveness is void. In some of the American painter Robert Ryman's large canvases, there is nothing – just white canvas.)

So what about Mondrian and his innumerable squares?

In serious cases of schizophrenia, the subject is first overwhelmed by the external world and cannot cope. He may then turn into himself for refuge, and fall back on basic abstract structures. Schizophrenics draw straight lines which express no emotional drive. Mondrian and others may not have been schizophrenics, but with their sensibility tuned to the era, they reveal the schizophrenic tendencies of our times.

The suicide of civilisation is reflected in that apparent return to realism which was Pop art – apparent because it was a realism of repulsion and contempt for the real. It can go quite far. In an exhibition a few years ago I saw a bottle containing a yellow liquid, and on the label, signed by the artist, was written 'This is my urine'. Have we not reached here the furthest point in that process of negation, sketched out by Picasso and developed by those who followed him? There has been a return to the real only to cancel it out and annihilate it.

## Contemporary art – the search for the spirit

After all this pessimism, let us now look at today's generation and its new openness. Many critics, fixed in their intellectual systems, do not understand it and accuse it of being a return to a realism already overtaken by modern art. I believe that young artists have assimilated the impact of abstract art and its structural sense and of surrealism and its plunge into the unspoken. But they have realised the need for a language of communication. As President of the Jury of the Grands Prix d'Art de Monaco, a competition for young people of thirty or forty at the oldest, each year I see works by young artists from all over the world. In the work of many of them a Neo-realism is apparent, not passive before nature, but one which borrows from nature a language to express the unspoken.

The winner of the Grand Prix in 1986, Richard Burtin, had a painting entitled *Pigeon mort* ('Dead pigeon') in which a distant influence of Mondrian could be detected in the assertive geometricisation of a window, as well as a return to the suggestive representation of the Surrealists. But the suggestion is no longer the same. It now comes from the shock of this dead bird placed under a window bursting with light and hope. Many other contemporary artists convey the same dualism of youth depressed with the dead end our civilisation has thrown it into, but at the same time silently longing for spiritual rebirth. *La fenêtre,* ('The window') (Figure 26.7) by Guy de Malherbe, another Monaco prizewinner in 1982, reveals a similar structure – abstract construction associated with the same profound meaning, expressed here by the young girl dressed in black – the spirit of youth reaching desperately out towards the light.

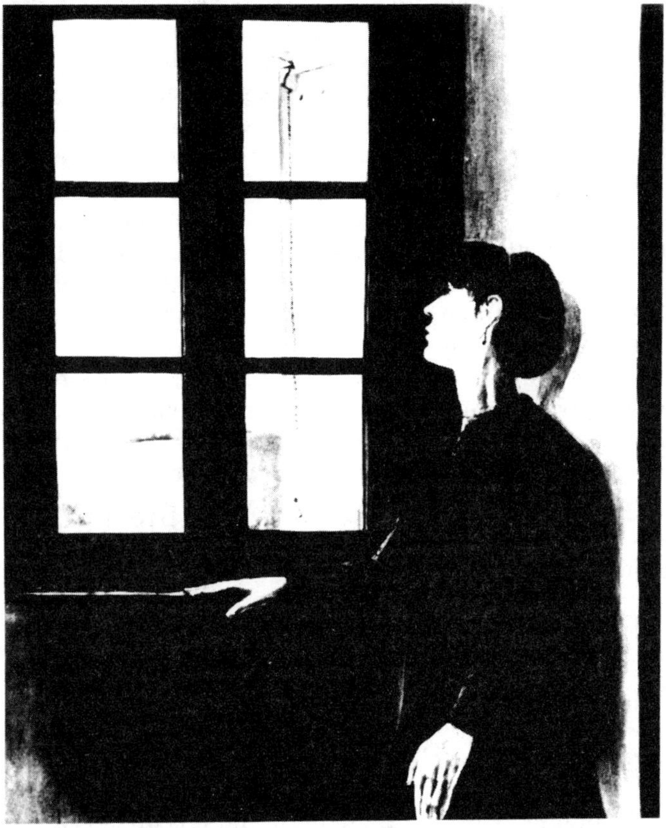

**Figure 26.7 Guy de Malherbe,** ***La fenêtre***

If we go back to Fred Zeller again, his *Chemin du ciel* ('Pathway to the sky') shows a typically melancholic figure sitting on the bottom steps of a flight of stairs to which it turns its back. But if we look closely, these steps lead to the sky and at the very top a torch is being lit. Can we not see in this the desire for a new spirituality?

In sculpture, the Austrian Henry Rosenthal creates, in *L'Escalade* ('The climb') a figure just as emaciated as Giacometti's, but his figure reaches up – desperately – for the sky, or perhaps heaven. Are these not the great eternal symbols that Jung studied in his archetypes? The spiritual quest is transformed, instinctively, into a struggle against the weight of matter. In all religions, levitation is a sign of saintliness, for saints, in their spiritual flight, cancel out their material weight. The flame which rises and gives light is another instinctive symbol: light is by essence immaterial, composed of photons and not atoms. Such archetypal symbols have always been present throughout the history of humankind, both in art and in literature.

Other contemporary painters and sculptors reveal the same archetypes – Lemaire d'Aggagio, in painting, or the greek sculptor Froso Eftimiadi.

This return to the spiritual had already been sketched out in some of the work of the surrealists, notably the Belgian René Magritte (1898–1967), whose painting *La grande famille* ('The great family') depicts the emptiness of the ocean and the sky, but with an immense bird taking flight. Through its exaggerated silhouette outlined against the sky, clear light appears. Similarly, in Max Ernst's 1958 painting *Après moi le sommeil* ('After me – sleep') we see a crystalline world building its shapes, while above the horizon a bird rises vertically.

Recently, while visiting the Italian painter Masini, I was struck by the fact that all his work was dominated by the obsession with birds flying in light, or through storms. He is typical of so many of the artists I have mentioned and many others – the subjects of their work are not the fruit of intellectual reflection, but rather of instinct. They carry a deep symbolic message to the rest of us, which it is for us to decode. This must be the only sure way, because what is wrong with our times is that all too often the intellectuals impose their reasonings and theories on painting, just as they do on society, instead of first letting the painters take the initiative and express themselves spontaneously. Then and only then should the intellectuals try to act as translators.

Science has studied matter's share of the universe. But the internal, subjective world has its share too and needs to be balanced against matter. The difference between the two is that in the physical world quantity rules, whereas in the internal world, it is quality. And it is precisely quality which puts morality in our acts, esthetics in our creations and, in the absolute, sets religions searching for God.

Chapter 27

# Efficiency and the pursuit of humanism

by Marianne Klees

Does not a society in which efficiency is a primary objective tend to neglect people's self-fulfilment and forget the pursuit of a certain humanism?[1]

Proud of their power, technocrats teach us that if we take account of the energy a person consumed and the techniques available to make work easier, a citizen of a rich country today 'is economically worth' eighty citizens from a developing country.

But as soon as we look at other criteria, we are faced with strikingly contrasting images.

- Well-fed American babies in hospitals, looked after with excellent health care, will go so far as to let themselves die through lack of affection, while babies in Bangladesh, clutched to their mothers' dried-up breasts, fight for survival;
- Genetic manipulation is used to modify chromosomes, but help for the handicapped is not universally considered as a criterion of civilisation;

---

[1] Humanism is any theory or doctrine whose concern is human beings and their fulfilment. It is a movement represented by the 'humanists' of the Renaissance and characterised by a desire to raise the dignity of, and give proper value to, the human mind.

- The computer will help to bring forward the age at which formal logic appears in children, and so help them to read, write and do mathematics, but the computer's magnetic memory does not know pity or leniency, and does not know how to excuse forgetfulness;
- There is a real explosion of psychological techniques to solve communication problems, but people, when they are together, only glance sideways at each other and, pushed for time (and time is money), talk less and less;
- In the industrialized world, education has become a 'pedagogical sprint' – children in Japan and the USA are crammed with learning techniques at an ever earlier age so as to have a head start over their toddler peers.

## Efficiency versus humanism

Each of the images above illustrates the capacity for power which we have gained through our efficiency – for better or for worse, for humanism or against it. And these images make us feel uneasy, guilty, humiliated by the contrast that exists between our extraordinary potential for creation, handed down and built upon from generation to generation, and our apparent inability to prevent this potential being used against humanity itself. Is not the root cause of this unease perhaps the pursuit of efficiency before all else?

Efficiency is a word which does not exist in the vocabulary of philosophy. It is a means and an action: obtaining the highest amount of useful work from the effort applied. It is the need for maximum productivity, especially in financial terms, but without taking account of the price paid by individuals who are more and more anonymous, depersonalised, lost in the mass. Efficiency is also integral to the transmission of doctrines, ideologies and slogans. The family, the clan, the tribe say loudly and clearly what we must think. Those who think they know take care to put their knowledge into dogma – for this is the quickest, most economical, surest and most efficient way of transmitting knowledge. The result is a potential domination and control of social conditions through 'organisations' which manage, dictate and implant value systems. This sort of efficiency is the opposite of free thinking and of humanism.

Humanism is that vision of the world which sees the human being as an end in itself. It defines its objectives through a system of ethical values. These are 'finalities of human actions defined in an abstract way by human beings who feel obliged to submit to them' (H. Jeanne). A value is an aspiration, felt collectively by a society or social group, which expresses a recognised truth in its social sphere. It concerns truth, goodness (what we should do and how), justice (rules of sharing, legitimisation of inequalities or equalities, equity in applying sanctions, and beauty (the esthetic aspect of all things and actions).

But it would not be useful, on principle, to offer efficiency and the pursuit of humanism as opposing alternatives. That would be to pose the problem in the wrong terms, to confuse the end and the means, the objective and strategies. This confusion is certainly a common error amongst certain planners and an easy temptation for decision-makers. It is especially an unacceptable abdication of responsibility for men and women of goodwill.

## The efficient pursuit of humanism

We need to rigorously reject all authoritarian argument – which by definition has no room for discussion – and develop a social and educational system based on dialogue. This is a demanding position to adopt – particularly in times of recession – because it restricts the flexibility of our response. We have to model our behaviour on the meaning and values we give to our lives, through our thinking (i.e. our way of perceiving reality intellectually) and through our actions (our way of influencing the outside world). Now more than ever we have to reconcile efficiency and humanism. The new alliance I am proposing is an efficiency which respects human beings and their dignity. Perhaps this is what we call 'competence', the competence we expect of people given the responsibility of governing, managing and teaching.

Efficient humanism is commitment to action, learning from mistakes, the strength which comes from fighting poverty and unhappiness. It is the evolution from fixed rules to a dialogue where the most competent listen to the less able and encourage them to speak as best they can. Out of this individuals will become lucid, open, rigorous, creative and ready for change. Efficiency in the pursuit of humanism is also the conquering of ignorance, educating people to examine and question accepted ideas and giving them the means of decoding biased information. And it is especially the encouragement of cross-disciplinary and cross-hierarchical exchange.

Some say that such an approach would complicate the organisation of work, and in the short term this might be true, for the complexity of human relationships requires a lot of energy, to the apparent detriment of productivity. But what would we think of a long-term profitability which resulted in a disinterested, faultless and humourless automation? Should not people be essential, losing neither their reality nor their ability to 'be', to feel and to think, and so develop their awareness and capacity for love?

## 'If Reason made Man, then Feeling drives him'

(J.-J. Rousseau)

Let us take together the first steps towards a society built of human complexity. To formal reasoning – where hypotheses and conclusions are articulated with an apparently undisputable coherence, so soundly are they based on logic – we need to add elements which are more intuitive, freer in their associations, less rigorous, and more 'real' because they come from us. These elements from ourselves, based on personal values, are necessarily different from one person to another, and hence are always open to discussion and to questioning according to each person's sensibility.

We need to let people speak and we need to listen to them – not to prove them right or wrong or to have the last word in a discussion, but to go down the same path together for a while. Seeing the world differently does not mean that the other person is lying. Let us listen to their answers to our questions and to the questions they ask. Without other people, without their eyes on us, their voices tingling our bones, guts and conscience, we are nothing. We fall, lose our way and crumble, buried, stupid, psychotic.

In his deeply symbolic book for children, *The Other*, André Chédid writes:

> Nuclear panoply, electronic marvels,
> Erasers of memories that hurt,
> Average lifespan 90 years, hibernation,
> Supercomputer ruling our lives,
> Community gobbling up the individual,
> Control, surveillance, telephonia,
> Materials resistant to any temperature,
> Propulsion transport, submergible cargos, container ships,
> Transoceanic rockets,
> Medicines controlling our moods, political tendencies, metaphysics,
> Determination of the sex of children,
> Synthesis of food,
> Pigmentation of Whites, depigmentation of Blacks,
> Detection of criminal intent from the sound of the voice,
> Superpower entente, quick and limited wars for the under-developed,
> Maelstrom, ... where, how to stay upright?
> Our defeat, do you know where it is?
>
> Perhaps in loving *things* more than the *way*.

Chapter 28

# The psychological roots of the environment crisis

by Peter Russell

The preceding papers in this book tell of the dangers facing us in terms of pollution, the toxicity of many of our products, the loss of our forests, electromagnetic pollution, the nuclear threat, the depletion of the ozone layer, and many other factors that threaten our health, and probably also our survival as a species. They also speak about the many changes that are needed in government policy, industrial practices, education, health care, and environmental management if we are to cope successfully with all these very real and very urgent issues. Certainly they need our fullest attention. But they are, I believe, all symptoms of a deeper, underlying problem.

Our lack of respect for Nature, our short-term thinking, and the damage we have caused to the biosystem are all symptoms of some deeper, underlying problem. We certainly need to clean up our act. But if we do not also look to the root cause of our inappropriate behaviours, then it is very possible that it will erupt in other symptoms.

What is the root of our environmental crisis? Why is it that one species out of millions has disrupted the natural balance in so many ways and with such dire consequences?

Let us look at the whole environmental issue in a much larger perspective. We are often so engrossed in our own particular period that we fail to see the full historical and evolutionary significance of the challenges we are currently facing.

It is, I believe, no exaggeration to say that we are living through the most exciting and challenging times ever in human history. Certainly there have been other very significant eras: the rise of the Egyptian culture, the Fall of Rome, the Renaissance and the Reformation, to name but a few – and to the people who lived through those periods they probably seemed to be the most significant ever. But none of these times carried the same implications for the future of humanity as do the closing days of the twentieth century.

These are times of unparalleled opportunity. The scientific and technological potentials are enormous. We have at our disposal the means to create the world almost any way we choose. Yet, despite these fantastic opportunities, the seeds of disaster are all around us. The very technology which gives us so much potential is also threatening our very existence. This may turn out to be the final period of human history.

Of all our technological achievements, the one that probably best characterises these times is our step out into space – a development which in evolutionary terms is probably as significant as the early amphibians' step from the sea onto land. We accomplished a dream almost as old as humanity itself. Not only did we push ahead the frontiers of technology and science, we also gained a new perspective of ourselves and planet Earth. For the first time we saw ourselves from the outside, and the view changed our thoughts and feelings in some unexpected ways.

For the early astronauts the sight of the planet floating in the blackness of space was a profound spiritual experience. One of them described it as 'instant global consciousness ... you are no longer an American citizen or a Russian citizen, suddenly all those boundaries disappear – you are a planetary citizen.'

The photographs of our planet brought back by the astronauts also had a profound effect on the rest of us (Figure 28.1). The picture here touches us in some deep way, as a result of which it has probably become the most common image in the world today. In some respects it is the spiritual symbol of our times. It symbolises the oneness of all humanity, and the oneness of all life on Earth. In this one image is reflected our whole concern for the planet and the fate of the human race.

Another realisation which struck some of the early astronauts was that, seen from a distance of a hundred thousand kilometres, the whole planet looked as if it might be some huge single living system. In a sense they were having a direct intimation of what has now become known as the Gaia Hypothesis, called after the Greek Earth goddess.

This theory suggests that the whole of the Earth's biosphere functions together as a single living system, maintaining the optimum conditions for its continued existence and evolution. The different species might be likened to the different organs in a body, each having its own function, and each supporting the functioning of the body as a whole. Of course the time-

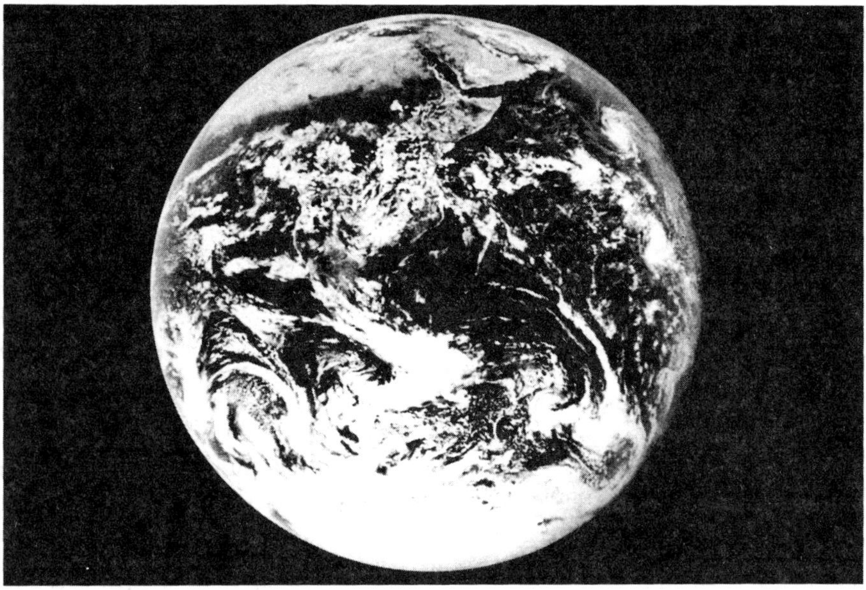

**Figure 28.1. A photograph of Earth brought back by American astronauts**

scales are very different, but the tropical rain forests might be seen as the liver, while the oceans and atmosphere perform, among other things, the function of a circulatory system. Our days and nights might be likened to the heart beat of the planet; and the seasons are more like her breaths.

But if the Earth is a living organism, what function do we play in it? Do we in fact play any useful function? The biosystem has, after all, survived quite well for several billion years without us. One possibility is that humanity is an embryonic global brain. Consider the ways in which telecommunications are linking us together across the planet, we find that there are indeed many parallels with the way the brain in an unborn child develops. Moreover, if the pace of development of information technology is sustained, it will only take a decade or two till our global telecommunications network equals the complexity of the human brain. Such a perspective has several interesting implications, which I have explored in more depth elsewhere.[1] But let us now consider another, far more sobering possibility: namely that humanity may be some form of planetary cancer.

---

1 Russell, P., *The Awakening Earth,* Ark, London, 1984, and Arkana, London, 1988; published in the USA as *The Global Brain,* Tarcher, Los Angeles, 1983.

## A planetary cancer?

Cancers can reproduce very fast, and without any regard for other organs. Cancer cells are essentially selfish cells, fulfilling their own needs at the expense of the organism as a whole. They are a part of the body, yet in many respects behave as if they were completely separate. They are also very stupid cells, destroying the very system on which their existence is totally dependent.

The parallels with humanity are not hard to see. Our population has been growing very rapidly, with little regard for the environment. Our own needs, or apparent needs, usually take precedence over those of our surroundings. We are a part of the biosphere and totally dependent upon it, yet we behave as if we were *apart* from the biosphere. We eat into the environment, eradicating natural ecosystems, spreading deserts of sand and concrete. We let our toxic wastes flow out into the environment, poisoning other species. Moreover, we too are very short-sighted, for if we continue, we may well destroy the biosystem, and hence ourselves.

Some believers in the Gaia hypothesis have suggested that if the planet does take care of herself, adjusting to changes in atmosphere, oceans and soil, so as to preserve the optimum conditions for continued life, then she will be able to adjust to humanity and evolve means to deal with our pollution and the other damage we have created. Our increased carbon dioxide output, for example, might be countered by an increase in marine micro-organisms which absorb the gas, leading back to a state of balance.

I believe such a view is dangerous for two reasons. Firstly, our rate of devastation is probably occurring over a much more rapid time-scale then Gaia can adjust to. But more importantly, the hypothesis suggests that the planet looks after her own welfare. She has no particular brief to preserve humanity. If we threaten the well-being of the Gaia, then perhaps the best thing she could do would be to get rid of us.

There are any number of ways in which she could do this. A nuclear war could be considered the Gaian equivalent of radiation treatment, although in both cases this should only be considered as a last resort since it tends to damage otherwise healthy parts of the body. We could wipe ourselves out with a bout of planetary chemotherapy – a nerve gas accident would do quite nicely. Or we could simply poison ourselves out of existence.

Or perhaps Gaia could summon her own immune response. Could AIDS be the response of the planet to a rather irritating species? It certainly would be a rather neat solution on her part: destroy the cancer without harming any other part of the system. Or is AIDS just a planetary warning shot across the bows? Perhaps we should be grateful that it is relatively difficult to spread. If AIDS had been as contagious as a common cold, then the whole of humanity would have been infected before we even knew the disease existed. Yet it is sobering to remember that the AIDS virus is evolving a hundred times faster than most other viruses, and may yet develop such virulence.

I do not wish to suggest that the healing of the planet necessitates the end of humanity. But if we are to avoid this rather depressing end, we must explore how we can rid ourselves of our own malignant tendencies. To see how this might be done and what it entails we need to look a little more deeply into the causes of our malignant attitudes.

## The roots of our crisis

In one way or another, the many crises which we face are all the result of decisions we have made. Evolution has blessed us with the faculty of choice and free will, and through them we have become active agents in the evolutionary process. But for one reason or another, we have frequently used this gift in ways which do not appear to support our own evolution or that of life as a whole.

The fact that we have not always chosen wisely suggests that the root of the error is not so much in our behaviour as in the thinking that underlies it, in the beliefs, values and criteria that underlie our thinking. The nuclear threat, the greenhouse effect, the destruction of the rain forests, the widescale extinction of species, acid rain, soil erosion, the depletion of the ozone layer, the problem of atomic waste, pollution, the energy crisis, the North-South crisis, the economic crisis, the food crisis, the water crisis, the housing crisis, the sanitation crisis, the AIDS crisis and all the many other crises that humanity faces are each symptoms of a deeper psychological crisis. Our motivations and goals are in some way inappropriate.

Again there are close parallels with cancer. In essence, cancer is an error of programming. In the heart of every cell are a set of chemical programmes, often loosely referred to as the genes, which contain instructions on how to build various complex proteins. These proteins underlie a cell's structure and behaviour. Although each cell in a body contains the same set of programmes, different parts are switched on for different cells and at different stages in the same cell's development. As a result, only a small proportion of the thousands of programmes in a particular cell are active at a given time.

Sometimes, however, sets of instructions which should be 'off' are switched on. This can happen for a number of reasons. Radiation from space, atomic waste or medical equipment may damage the control sequences – the switches in the gene. Toxic chemicals in the air, in water or in food, may damage the programmes. Or a virus may enter the cell and replace the genetic material with some of its own.

Often the results are benign. But sometimes the cell may begin growing and reproducing itself. Guided by a set of instructions totally inappropriate to its natural function in the body, it becomes a 'selfish', rogue cell no longer acting in harmony with rest of the body. This is the beginning of cancer.

Likewise humanity's malignant tendencies could be considered to stem from errors of programming. In this case the programmes are our attitudes, beliefs and values; our basic operating principles; the mind sets we have about who we are and what is important.

We may take the attitude that our own benefit comes before that of others. We may believe that we can own the land, own the planet's natural resources and even own other lifeforms. We may value our material possessions more for the status they give than for their utility. We may think that we can become happy through accumulating personal wealth. Since the choices we make – both individually and collectively – are conditioned by our attitudes and values, it is little wonder that we use our creativity and technology in ways which benefit us only in the short term (and even this is questionable). It would appear that the roots of humanity's malignancy lie deep within our minds, at the very heart of our functioning.

Our decisions are driven by the needs we perceive. We have various physical needs – air, food, water, warmth, shelter; we have various psychological needs – belonging, recognition, security, control, stimulus. Most, although not all, people living in the more developed countries have their physical needs met; indeed, one of the goals of social development is the adequate fulfilment of these needs. What drives us, then, is our psychological needs.

The need for security, for example, often manifests itself as the need for wealth, although money also offers a sense of status. Much of our social behaviour is geared towards gaining the approval and recognition of others. The foods we choose to eat are often chosen more for their ability to stimulate the taste buds than their nutritional value; and if they can be consumed in up-market restaurants, we gain an added psychological boost.

Unfortunately, however, whereas our physical needs can be satisfied, our psychological needs are rarely fulfilled. A person may gather a great deal of wealth, but does he feel more secure as a result? He then finds new sources of insecurity. Others may try to steal his wealth, and he has to employ 'security' companies to defend his accumulated riches. Or you may discover the gastronomic excellence or sexual ecstasy you have been seeking for years. Does this then satisfy you? Or are you left wondering when you might be able to repeat the experience? It seems that we have become stuck with various needs that are not really necessary.

Some have argued that human beings have a hardware fault. Somewhere in our evolution our brains have been 'mis-wired', with the result that we are born with an inherently selfish, aggressive and competitive nature. But I want to suggest the likelihood that it may in fact be a software problem – an error in our programming. In this case there may be hope for humanity, for perhaps the error can be corrected. But to know whether or not this is possible, we must first ask why we hold on to our psychological needs so strongly. What underlies our psychological needs?

## The search for identity

The answer, I believe, lies in one of our deepest psychological needs – our survival programming. The urge to maintain one's physical integrity is very natural and is found in all creatures. Yet human beings also have an urge to maintain their sense of psychological integrity – their sense of self and personal identity.

Most people's primary sense of identity is derived from their experience and interaction with the world. I 'am' my personality, my character, my job, my social status, my sex, my body, my nationality, my name, my family, my ideals, my beliefs, my education, my interests, my clothes and even, sometimes, my car. None of these are really who 'I' am; they are things we have or do, things that describe us and identify us to others. They are how the 'I' is seen rather than the essence of 'I'.

But if this is our only sense of identity we are stuck in a trap. For when one of the things from which we derive our outer identity changes or is threatened, our sense of identity is threatened. The result is that we spend a considerable amount of time and energy on protecting, maintaining and defending this outer identity. The net effect is that we come to love things more than our own being.

If this were as far as it went, such sad and unnecessary behaviour would be benign. But its consequences spread out into the world around. We end up exploiting the world around in service of this partial sense of self – and 'the world around' includes other people as well as our physical and biological environment. Our need for recognition and approval can lead us to make inappropriate political, economic, environmental or industrial decisions. Our need to defend our beliefs can turn others into enemies, make us kill *en masse* and focus half our technology on weapons of war. Over-concerned with our psychological survival, we consume resources we do not need, disperse toxins we could contain and carelessly eliminate many of the other species who share this planet with us.

We often think of big business as the exploiters of nature; but we are all exploiters in one way or another, and we are all to blame for the crisis in which we find ourselves. We can certainly legislate to some effect, but the very nature of legislation means that it is nearly always in conflict with some individual's needs; if it were not, it would hardly be necessary.

So we see that humanity's problem is that it has become riddled with self-centredness. Its is as if the minds of humanity are diseased with a mental virus called 'ego'. And this mental virus poses a far more dangerous threat than does the AIDS virus. For it is this self-centredness that governs our attitudes, that keeps us locked into behaviour that is neither for own good nor that of the planet, and that often prevents us from making the very changes in our behaviour that we know are so essential.

## An evolutionary perspective

This problem of egocentricity seems to be uniquely human. The great apes do not seem to have egos that need continual reinforcement. Why is that we do? And why in ways that are so obviously damaging to our own long-term interests?

The answer probably goes back to the two things that most distinguish us from all other creatures. The first is our highly developed symbolic language. Among other things, language gave us the ability to describe and define our experience. This has led to science, understanding, communication, caring and the evolution of human culture. Without the many spin-offs that language gave us, we would never have evolved to the stage where we are now. But there are possible pitfalls to giving too much value to language.

So successful is language in its ability to describe and define that we unwittingly make the assumption that everything can be described and defined. Through language we are able to throw more light on the world, but can we throw light onto the self, which is the source of the light? However much we try to grasp the self in words or concepts, we fail to find the source of our experience. And we may well conclude, as many have done, that there is some mystery at play, or that there is no such thing as the self. But we are still aware.

Crucial as language may have been in the evolution of human society, it has little value when it comes to knowing our true identity. All that can be described of ourselves are the aspects of our being that can be experienced, either by us or by others. Thus in trying to define ourselves to ourselves, we all too easily come to identify ourselves with our outer selves, the self that can be seen.

In itself this limited identity may not have serious consequences for the rest of humanity. Many of the materially less developed societies seem to have successfully integrated the needs of the ego with the needs of the group. The consequences start to become serious when this derived sense of self is combined with the other feature which distinguishes us from all other creatures – our opposable thumbs.

This unique feature allows us to grasp objects of varying shapes and sizes, manipulate them, and perform delicate operations with them. Combine this beautiful evolutionary advance with a brain able to think, gather knowledge and contemplate the future, and you have a creature able to make a rich variety of tools – hammers, axes, spears, clothes, boats, wheels, windmills, steam engines, telephones, computers and space vehicles. The whole of human technology can be seen as the amplification of the power inherent in the human thumb.

Technology has amplified our ability to influence and change the world for our ends, and in ways far beyond the capacities of any other creature. If those ends are important for our survival and welfare as a species, then technology could be a great asset. When, however, the ends are those of an identity which continually seeks to change the world in order to reinforce its sense of individual existence, then technology can become very dangerous to all concerned. In the words of the late Gregory Bateson:

> If this is your estimate of your relationship to nature, and you have a high technology, your likelihood of survival will be that of a snowball in hell. You will die either of the toxic by-products of your own hate, or simply of over-population and over-grazing. The whole of our thinking about who we are has got to be restructured.

In other words high technology and an under-evolved psyche cannot coexist for long. One of them must go. There is little chance of technology disappearing – and few would want it to. It is our psyches that must change. The ego must go.

## The consciousness crisis

At its root, then, the crisis of our times is not so much an environmental crisis, an economic crisis, a population crisis or a political crisis; it is in essence a consciousness crisis – a mismatch between our psychological development and our technological development. We do not yet have the inner wisdom and freedom to use our new powers for the good of all.

We should not necessarily judge ourselves badly for falling out with Nature in this way. It may well be a temporary, but inevitable, phase in the evolution of an intelligent species that develops both technology and a sense of self. If dolphins had had fingers and thumbs, they might well have had to face a similar psychological crisis.

This consciousness crisis probably comes upon an intelligent species very quickly. As soon as it emerges from the biological phase of its evolution into its cultural phase, a species is engaged in a dash through history. The dash begins with the emergence of self-reflective consciousness and ends in the species' consciousness crisis. As the species rapidly evolves, it develops the means of its own demise. And as its development accelerates, it brings the testing point ever closer.

As a species we are facing our final examination right now. It is a psychological examination, in fact a test of our true intelligence as a species. The question that has been set is very simple: Are we as a species able to use the awesome power we have developed for the good of the Universe?

In essence we are being asked to let go of our self-centred thinking and egocentric behaviour. We are being asked to become psychologically mature, to free ourselves from the clutches of this limited identity and to express our creativity in ways which benefit us all.

This test is not just being posed to governments, corporations and scientific institutions; it is being posed to all of humanity. Can we each personally realise that our real identity is not dependent upon the things we gather around us, the way others see us, or the way we like to see ourselves?

Can we realise that the ego-mode is not the only mode, and certainly no longer the most appropriate? And can we then release ourselves from its grip, and allow our true intelligence to shine into the world?

We know this shift is possible for we have seen many examples of people who have lived it – the St Theresas, the St Francises and all the other saints, whether they be called saints or just simple people. We know inside that this is how life can be lived and should be lived, but somehow we feel it is too far away or not for us. Or we are too caught up in the world, with no time to spare. Or we feel trapped in other ways.

But we also know that it is not beyond us. Many of us have at times felt what it means to be simply oneself, secure in one's own existence. It may have been triggered by a beautiful sunrise, through falling in love, during meditation, or in a confrontation with death. Suddenly the mind falls back into its natural state, a state of ease.

What we do not know is how to allow this ease to fall upon us. We are so caught up in all the things that we believe we need, we never allow time to let it be.

Perhaps we need the psychological equivalent of the Manhattan Project. That was the code word for the development of the first atomic bomb. It had been realised that in the new found energies of the atomic nucleus was the potential to release vast amounts of energy. Initiating a chain reaction could create a bomb a thousand times more powerful than the high explosives of the day. The development of such a bomb was seen to be of the highest importance for ending World War II, and hence for global security. Consequently, scientific, technical and financial resources were pumped into a number of research and development institutions across the

United States. The result was the detonation, within less than three years, of the first atomic bomb.

Now, nearly fifty years later, it is becoming clear that there are enormous untapped potentials within human consciousness, the nucleus of our being. If this power can be released, humanity could begin to tackle its problems much more wisely, ending the possibility of world war and greatly increasing our chances of survival. If this need were recognised and resources were put into projects to explore how to facilitate our awakening, then we could have an Inner Manhattan Project, one of far greater value than the original. The Manhattan Project was founded to win a war against other people; this Inner Manhattan Project would help us win the war against ourselves.

The wisdom of the human psyche already exists in many spiritual traditions, philosophies and psychologies. But it needs to be pulled together and researched in order to bring out the essential wisdom in a manner which the person in the street can recognise and claim. This is not to advocate a return to religions of the past, but a rediscovery of the sacred within us in the language and technologies of the twentieth century.

We might liken humanity to a person who has fallen ill. A doctor who merely gave the person ointments, pain relievers and something to suppress the temperature would not be considered very wise. Clearly, true healing requires that, in addition to treating the various symptoms, one must also look more deeply at what underlies them. Perhaps a foreign bacteria is present; maybe there is vitamin deficiency; or possibly the person's emotional state is responsible. If the roots of the symptoms are not also treated, then it is almost certain that the illness will reappear, possibly in other forms.

Similarly with humanity. Any lasting remedy must seek to find the underlying cause of the malady. Certainly we need to do everything we can to reduce the damage we are causing to the environment. But if this is all that we do, we shall find the same illness reappearing in other symptoms.

I have argued that the root of the environment crisis lies deep within our psyches – in our sense of identity, our needs, our attitudes and our values. It is, in essence, a spiritual crisis. Environmental science already includes many of the physical and biological sciencies within its scope. A truly holistic approach must, however, include the psychological sciences and have the courage to explore the deeper spiritual issues behind the crisis. It may sound unorthodox and it may not be easy; but it is, I believe, our only hope.

# Part V

# Appendix

# The conference poster sessions

by Antonius F. W. Morselt

While the papers and discussions at the conference **Man...Health... Environment** were concerned with the general principles of environmental health, the poster sessions concentrated on current research in the field. There was a great diversity of subjects displayed because the environment approaches us in so many ways and is studied by so many different disciplines – chemists, biologists, medical doctors, engineers, architects, etc.

Several posters dealt with projects in areas where ecotoxicology intersects with human health, i.e. where the different constituents of soil, water and air have impacts on nature and human health. G. De Mets, of the Belgian Building Research Institute, studied radon concentrations in houses. Radon concentration can be dangerous for human health when it measures above 200 becqerels per cubic metre. Based on a survey of certain regions in Belgium, De Mets found a high radon concentration only in houses in those villages where the soil has a high radium content. He recommended that both remedial and preventive action be taken against this hidden danger.

Dr J.A. Aten of the University of Amsterdam presented an ingenious method to detect precancerous damage of chromosomes. This work is of particular importance because low levels of radiation can give rise to cancer after a number of years.

Dr B. Jeppesen studied the relationship between ischemic heart diseases and drinking water. He found that the water in Greenland is extremely soft and that the calcium/magnesium ratio in the blood of the Greenlanders is significantly lower than in the blood of the Danes. Even though Greenlanders lead the same stressful, westernized life as the Danes these days, his study reported, Greenland has one-third to one-sixth fewer cases of ischemic heart disease than Denmark.

Professor I. Rigo reported research showing an increase in free magnesium in Hungarian soil due to acidification. This occurrence could also show up in drinking water and may be connected to the occurrence of ischemic heart disease in Hungary.

A mutagenicity test to measure the effects of pollutants in drinking water on human genetic material was introduced by Dr L. Hens of the Free University of Brussels. An increased mutagenicity implies an increased risk to cancer. The test provides a useful biological indicator of potentially harmful groundwater that chemical methods cannot detect.

Dr A.F.W. Morselt of the University of Amsterdam drew attention to 'therapies' against the damage to plants and trees caused by acid rain derived from the soil compartment. Nowadays, in many regions of Europe the metal content in the soil is much above normal. His research showed that by making mycorrhiza (fungi which live in symbiosis with nearly all plants and trees) resistant to heavy metals, new seedlings innoculated with these fungi have a possibility of surviving in metal-polluted areas. Dr Morselt recommended that governments stimulate research to develop other possible therapeutic approaches to acid rain that can be derived from the soil compartment.

Pollutants in water can also influence the health of fish species. J.R. Grezes of Schallstadt (FRG) demonstrated that industrial dyes cause risks to fish health and reproduction. Dr P.W. Wester, of the Dutch National Institute of Public Health and Environmental Protection of Holland (RIVM), showed that by using histopathology on a very small fish (e.g. a guppy), the toxicity of various kinds of pollutants in the water can be predicted more accurately. Dr D. de Zwart of the same institute developed a test to establish the chemically induced disturbance of interactions between functionally different groups of organisms in a model ecosystem – algae, daphnids, polyps and decomposer organisms respectively.

Two posters dealt with pollutants in the air. Dr E. Dimitrescu of the University of Paris showed convincing evidence on the correlation between asthma attacks and the quantity of sulphur dioxide in the centre of Paris. Her results might imply that people who have a genetic predisposition to asthma which is not derived from known allergens should live in less polluted areas.

In an experimental animal study, Dr H. van Loveren of RIVM established that ozone, given together with a bacterial infection, caused a suppression in the cellular immune defence of the lungs.

Governments need and use methods of risk assessment for environmental pollutants. Dr A. Steenhout of the Free University of Brussels proposed a new method of risk assessment for lead which considers all the lead fluxes from the sources of emissions to the various human tissues. She claims the new method is superior in certain respects to that now being used by the European Communities.

According to studies presented by Dr M. Mansour of the Institute of Ecological Chemistry, Munich, some pollutants in the air require less or no remedial action. He has found that a number of chemical substances undergo abiotic degradation by sunlight or oxygen before they enter the human organism.

Some posters showed findings that human health is also affected by extra-terrestrial environmental influences. Dr D.M. Mikhov of the Institute of Neurology, Sofia, showed a correlation between suicide attempts and different moon phases in a study that covered 9,000 participants and lasted eight years. Moreover, he found both that suicide attempts increase significantly on days with geomagnetic storms and that season also seems to have an influence.

## *Environmental pollutants and civilisation diseases*

The relationship between environmental pollutants and civilisation diseases – i.e. those occurring predominantly after the industrial revolution – was the theme of many of the posters. Dr A. Peretz, of the University Hospital, Brussels, presented a multidisciplinary study of osteoporosis (a weakening of the bone tissue), which in Western countries affects more than twenty-five per cent of the female population aged over forty-five. The study covered a group of 2,246 women and identified a number of external risk factors, sich as certain nutritional factors (low calcium intake, high protein intake, high coffee intake, lactose intolerance, alcohol intake), endocrine factors related to meno- and andropause, stress, drug use, race and physical activities.

There are several theories about the causes of Alzheimer disease – a mental threat to our modern society. Dr G.V. van der Voet of the University of Leiden presented evidence for the relationship between neurological disorders and the ubiquitous occurrence of aluminium in the environment. His investigations showed an increase of aluminium intestinal absorption if citrate was used in the diet.

It is known that disturbances in lipid metabolism lead to arteriosclerosis and myocardial infarction. Dr M Popischil of the University Clinic for

Industrial Medicine, Vienna, studied the relation between lipid metabolism and long-term exposure to low levels of organic solvents used in a number of jobs. He found that the solvents did not disturb the lipid metabolism; instead it seemed that nutritional habits were the most important factors causing such disturbance.

Different temperatures in the indoor climate of a workplace can improve or reduce productivity, according to studies done by Dr L. Pöllmann of the University of Giessen. He also demonstrated how heat and cold can be used to treat or prevent some diseases. For example, he found that warm/cold foot baths in a curative dosage led to resistance against infections of the common cold.

Relatively few studies have been performed on differences in individual susceptibility towards environmental pollutants. In his investigations in this area, Dr A.F.W. Morselt used an animal model and cell biology techniques. His studies suplied a number of explanations for the differences in susceptibility towards the environmental pollutant cadmium and found that the factor of genetic constitution with its related parameters seems especially important.

Most people living in European climates spend a great deal of time in their homes; thus indoor climate and atmosphere are important factors in their health and architects have an important role to play in environmental health. Professor P. Schmid, of the Technical University of Eindhoven, presented the philosophy of integral biological architecture. Architect R.J. Dietrich of Munich showed how this type of architectural philosophy was used in a number of house designs fulfilling health requirements. His most striking example is called the super-igloo, a model of which will soon be constructed in the Munich area. For cases where environmental accidents require the quick re-housing of large numbers of people, I.O. Szorady, a Budapest architect, has developed an ingenious high-technology shelter which can be used in all types of climate.

Mrs Garrity of the Institution of Environmental Health Officers, London, showed how this non-governmental organisation plays a leading role in promoting environmental health in the United Kingdom. It gives education and training to around 6,000 environmental health officers employed by local authorities, publishes documents and also organises campaigns.

Nowadays health problems caused by environmental pollution is worked on by researchers coming from different scientific disciplines. Dr J. Kleinjans showed how the University of Limburg (NL) is developing a full-scale academic programme in environmental health sciences that would graduate professionals specially trained for the field.

## *Philosophical overview*

Professor J.W. Dobrowolski of the University of Krakow presented a philosophical overview of the current state of environmental research. He pointed out that fragmentary research in this field is being carried out in nearly all parts of the globe. These piecemeal studies cost a great deal of money, yet they are contributing relatively little to the practice of environmental health. Prof. Dobrowolski proposed various general ways of channelling and guiding these investigations towards more realistic health problems.

It is reassuring, in a way, that thanks to modern analytical equipment this research can be done and the public is becoming more aware of the different threats to health. But we must still question whether adequate environmental health measures are being taken in each country and whether the limited resources available are being put to the best use.

It is very difficult to choose which types of studies should be given priority. Does the risk of cancer derived from drinking water take priority over the risk of cancer derived from radiation? Most of the posters described here represented different fields of environmental research, each with its own value for the health of humans and the ecosystem.

Most investigators communicate well with others in their same special field of environmental research. But as we were shown by the conference, environmental health is an area which calls upon scientists in the natural and social sciences to break out of their own categories and to approach problems in a holistic way.

Just as significant is the communication gap between individual researchers in the various areas of environmental health and those who formulate and take the decisions for environmental measures. A small, practical step forward might be the scheduling of regular, well-planned discussion groups between politicians, civil servants and rotating members of the scientific research community. Perhaps through such improved communication we will be able to begin to piece together the real dimensions and implications of the dangers which mankind has brought – and continues to bring – upon the health of humans and the ecosystem.

*(The posters presented at the conference were submitted by the researchers and represent only a small sample of the many studies currently being done on the different aspects of environmental health. Further information about the studies mentioned can be obtained from the researchers, who are listed below.)*

Aten, J., *Automatic detection by flow cytometry of chromosome aberrations induced by radiation or chemical agents.* Laboratory for Radiobiology, University of Amsterdam, Meibergdreef 9, NL-1105 AZ Amsterdam.

De Mets, G., *The influence of uranium soil on radon concentration in dwellings* and *Natural radioactivity in Belgian dwellings.* Belgian Building Research Institute, Lombardstraat 41, B-1000 Brussels.

De Zwart, D., *Chemically induced community responses in a compartmentalized microcosm assessed by state-space transitions.* RIVM, P.O. Box 1, NL-3720 BA Bilthoven.

Dietrich, R.J., *Ecological architecture.* Adelbertstrasse 55, D-8000 Munich 40.

Dumitrescu, E., *Impact of the urban environment and of atmospheric pollution on human health.* Université de Paris I Sorbonne, 2ter Rue Broussais, F-Paris 75014.

Dobrowolski, J.W., *Scientific premises for the anticipation of health hazards associated with deterioration of the human environment.* Institute of Management and Environment Protection, 30-059, Krakow, al. Mickiewicza 30, POL-Paw. C-4, Poland.

Garrity, *A concept of modern education for improving the quality of the human environment.* c/o Mrs Battersby, The Institution of Environmental Health Oficers, Chadwick House, Rushworth Street, UK-London SE1 0QT.

Grezes, J.R., *An ecotoxicological study of effects of industrial dyes on fish species.* Laboratoire Privé, Baslerstrasse 93, D-7801 Schallstadt.

Hens, L., *The use of the SCE test in human lymphocytes to test monitoring well water samples from polluted soils.* Vrije Universiteit Brussel, Pleinlaan 2, B-1050 Brussels.

Jeppesen, B., *Greenland: soft-water area – ischemic heart death – calcium/magnesium ratio.* Saeby Sygehus, Tjornelundevej 17, Tjornelunde, DK-4270 Hong, Sjaelland, Denmark.

Kleinjans, J., *Design of a full-scale graduation programme in environmental health sciences.* Department of Human Biology, University of Limburg, P.O. Box 616, NL-6200 MD Maastricht.

Mansour, M., *The significance of abiotic degradation in evaluation of persistent pollutants in the environment.* Institut für Ökologische Chemie, D-8050 Freising-Attaching.

Mikhov, D., *External physical factors and human behaviour,* and *Moon phases and attempted suicide by poisoning.* Institute of Neurology, Psychiatry and Neurosurgery, Lenin Boulevard 4th Km, 1113 Sofia, Bulgaria.

Morselt, A.F.W., *Why is one individual more susceptible for cadmium toxicity than another? Some answers by using cell biology methods,* and *A possible 'therapy' against the damage to forest by acid rain using induction of metallothionein in ectomycorrhizal fungi.* Laboratory for Histology and Cell Biology, University of Amsterdam, Academic Medical Centre, Meibergdreef 15, NL-1105 AZ Amsterdam.

Peretz, A., *Age dependency of bone remodelling parameters in the assessment of osteoporosis: an epidemiological study,* and *Multidisciplinary approach for the study of osteoporosis by the organisation of a data bank.* Rheumatology Department, Hôpital Universitaire St. Pierre, 322 Rue Haute, B-1000 Brussels.

Pöllman, L., *Opinions on a constant indoor climate,* and *A thermophysiological approach to the common cold.* Institut und Poliklinik für Arbeits- und Sozialmedizin der Universität, Aulweg 129/III, D-6300 Giessen.

Pospischil, M., *Is there an influence of long-term exposure to organic solvents at low levels on lipid metabolism?* Universitätsklinik für Arbeitsmedizin, Spitalgasse 23, A-1090 Vienna.

Rigo, J., *Changes in magnesium content of the soil in Hungary.* The National Institute of Dietetics, H-1085 Budapest VIII, Makarenkó u. 24, Hungary.

Schmid, P., *Healthy building in detail.* Technische Universiteit Eindhoven, P.O. Box 513, NL-5600 MB Eindhoven.

Steenhout, A., *The ecotoxicological causality analysis for lead exposure risk assessment.* Institut de Pharmacie, Université Libre de Bruxelles, P.O. Box 205/6, B-1050 Brussels.

Szórády, I.O., *Shelter for the homeless! A high-tech shelter system to be built for catastrophe or poverty stricken areas.* H-1124 Budapest, Vas Greben u. 32.1.5, Hungary.

Van der Voet, G., *Intestinal absorption and systematic transport of aluminium: relation to neurotoxicity.* Toxicology Laboratory, University Hospital Leiden, NL-2300 RC Leiden.

Van Loveren, H., *Effect of ozone exposure on defence to respiratory infection in the rat.* Laboratory for Pathology, RIVM, P.O. Box 1, NL-3720 BA Bilthoven.

Wester, P.W., *Histopathology of* P. Reticulata *(Guppy) and* O. Latipes *(Medaka) in toxicity testing of some environmental contaminants.* RIVM, P.O. Box 1, NL-3720 BA Bilthoven.